Ketogenic Diet:

The Complete Guide to Losing Weight on the Keto Diet for Beginners. Includes Simple Keto Reset Diet Recipes + 4 Week Meal Prep Plan. Live Longer, Be Healthier, and Transform Your Life

Randall Colbert

Table of Contents

Conclusion...113

Introduction

Congratulations on downloading *Ketogenic Diet* and thank you for doing so.

If you have downloaded this book, then you are probably curious about the keto diet. This diet has become very popular in recent years because of the astonishing weight loss results it produces. Not just that, it's been known to improve overall health and help at-risk diabetes or heart disease patients. This makes the keto diet a sustainable, long-term diet plan to improve your health. The keto diet is a unique one because it requires a majority intake of high-quality fat, a moderate intake of protein, and very minimum carbohydrate intake—75% fat, 20% protein, and ~5% carbohydrates. That's because eating carbohydrates tends to cause blood sugar spikes and create glucose molecules for energy. With the reduction of carbohydrates and increase in fat, we hope to harness energy through the process of ketosis which produces ketones, or rich energy molecules composed of fat. This means you are burning the fat reserves you have stored away which helps you lose weight and actually gives you more energy and better concentration.

This book is here to help beginners learn why the keto diet is highly recommended and the successful results it produces. From learning about what ketosis is and how to push your body towards this physiological process to learning about the benefits and drawbacks of keto, you can decide about whether keto is right for you. If you have medical issues or history with an eating disorder, you should not start this diet. Before making any changes to your lifestyle, it's important that you first speak with your physician to ensure the keto diet would be helpful for you. Whether you're hoping to lower your blood pressure, shed weight, or lessen the possibility of having diabetes, this diet can help you improve your health and see results.

With successful tips on how to get started on keto and what mistakes to avoid, this book also provides more than 30 easy-to-make keto recipes for breakfast, lunch, dinner, and dessert! That's right, we will even help you satisfy your sweet tooth cravings with delicious and keto-friendly snacks. By assisting you with your keto shopping list and clearly laying out what you can and cannot buy, you'll feel more confident as you shop for your meals and plan for the week ahead. We help you meal plan upcoming meals so you can save time, money, and the headache of what to eat!

We hope this book will give you a thorough understanding of keto and exactly how this diet has helped millions of people achieve better health and lose stubborn body fat. With plenty of information on what you can and cannot eat and the healthy and delicious recipes with dietary information, you are ready to embark on a keto diet and change your life today!

A lot of books on this subject are on the market, so thanks again for choosing this one! Every effort was made to ensure it is full of as much useful information as possible. Please enjoy!

Chapter 1: What Is the Keto Diet?

The Keto Diet, Ketones, and Ketosis

The ketogenic diet, or keto for short, has swept the nation in recent years. Why? Because it works! Millions of people have followed this diet and seen weight loss results and improved their overall health. This diet follows a regiment where a person's daily intake of carbohydrates remains very low to drive the body towards a state of ketosis.

Usually, most people's diets consist of nearly 70% carbohydrates. When the body is consuming carbohydrates, the stomach breaks down the food and creates sugar molecules called glucose. This is the easiest and quickest molecule of energy for the body to produce to give us instant energy. Glucose can either be used immediately by the body or be transported and stored as energy. The problem is that when glucose stays in the bloodstream, it causes blood sugar levels to become high, which can be a sign of trouble for diabetic or borderline diabetes patients. The pancreas then secretes insulin which is used to transport glucose throughout the bloodstream. The secretion of insulin is triggered by beta cells in the bloodstream. For example, if you eat something high in carbohydrates, like a piece of bread or a pastry, glucose levels will rise in the bloodstream. To counteract this, the beta cells will trigger the pancreas to produce more insulin into the bloodstream to carry the glucose away. That's why having too many carbohydrates can be dangerous for a diabetes patient because it causes the level of insulin to skyrocket.

So, how does the keto diet affect this phenomenon for the better? This diet has shown to make significant decreases in insulin and blood sugar levels for patients at risk of diabetes or who have diabetes. With the addition of losing weight and other multiple health benefits, it's natural to see why this diet has become so popular for diabetic patients to control their blood sugar!

A standard keto diet will follow a macronutrients breakdown that is low in carbs, high in fat, and with a moderate amount of protein. Macronutrients are referred to primarily as the large building blocks of your diet where your energy comes from. The breakdown will usually be:

75% fat
20% protein
~5% carbohydrates

The carbohydrate intake is usually recommended to stay around 20-30 grams. That means net carbs which is what you're left with after subtracting the fiber from the total carbohydrates per serving. For example, if you're eating something that has 20 grams of carbohydrates total, but with 6 grams fiber, your net carbohydrates intake for that food item would be 14 grams. This can often cause confusion with beginners, so that's why it's very important when first starting the keto diet to keep track of your carbohydrate intake. That allows you to track your individual macros and ensure you aren't going over your daily breakdown. If you find you're not losing weight as you anticipated on the keto diet, it could be a beginner's mistake where you aren't keeping track of your diet and are maybe eating too many carbs or too much protein. Having the correct balance in your diet breakdown and minimizing your carbohydrates intake is what will push your body into ketosis which will allow you to lose weight and gain the health benefits.

This diet can be changed slightly depending on a person's individual needs. For example, athletes might need extra carbohydrates intake for fuel before their workout so they will need a more specific keto diet which increases their carbs. We will talk about the more individualized keto diet types in the next chapter.

When you are on keto and you are consuming a higher fat content and a lower carbohydrates intake, your body cannot make glucose the usual way. It has to switch to a new process to make fuel. This new metabolic process to make energy is called "ketosis". When you are eating high-quality fats as the keto diet demands, you are pushing your body to burn fat for energy instead of carbohydrates. The liver begins to convert the fatty acids from your diet into molecules called "ketones". This is an alternative form of energy than glucose, but a more efficient one because it provides more energy per molecule. Glucose is the "quick" method of the body making fuel, while ketones are made of higher-quality fat to provide more sustained energy. By burning these "ketones" of fat for energy, the body can lose weight more efficiently. It's using the fat it had stored away as a reserve instead of constantly burning through the carbohydrates you are eating to fuel the body.

There are some critics of the keto diet who say that pushing the body towards a state of ketosis by depriving it of carbohydrates is unnatural and a drastic move to reduce weight. But human evolution tells us that's not true at all! Our bodies were created to have multiple pathways to harness energy from the food we are eating. The reason we follow the glucose producing pathway so often is that we have naturally gravitated towards diets high in carbohydrates. If that's how we've trained our bodies, then that is how they will respond based on what we are eating. When you change the content of your diet, your body is armed with natural receptors that recognize a shortage in carbohydrates. It doesn't panic; it just realizes it needs to create energy in a different pathway, so it begins the process of ketosis. Think about how primitive societies would have adapted to famine or stress factors if their body could not naturally adjust. When shortages in the food supply would occur, societies would naturally minimize their diet or begin to fast to save the food for the elderly or children in the community. Their bodies would not shut down; they would simply adjust and create energy in another way. It would harness energy from the fats it had already stored away as a reserve and use those to create immediate fuel as necessary.

It's the same parallel if you were trying to quit smoking or caffeine from your diet. Your body has become dependent on a substance, but it was not created that way from the very beginning. It had to make that change and adjust, just like you will have to make the motivational change to quit for health reasons. The same goes for carbohydrates! If a person is at a detrimental health risk of high blood sugar, then it's important they adjust their diet by cutting back on their carbohydrate intake. Following the keto diet allows them to provide their body with an alternative pathway for energy.

Carbohydrates, Sugars, and Ketones

Carbohydrates are still an important food group that provides us with quick, instant energy. There's a reason why it has become more than half of our daily diet—it works, and it's delicious! It's the only fuel that releases its energy without oxygen, so it is essential in a life-or-death situation where you, all of a sudden, are short of breath and need the energy to run or flee. Or even when you are working out and need that last push of energy to complete your training.

But the problem becomes when people are eating too many carbohydrates and having too much glucose in their system. That can increase your risk of obesity, diabetes, and other diseases. Instead of gaining fuel and energy, you're becoming more unhealthy! If you have a consistently high intake of carbohydrates, your body will actually store it as extra fat! This becomes a cyclical process—you may try to work out and get rid of that stubborn fat, but if you are eating an unhealthy diet that contains too many carbs, your body will continue to store it as fat reserves. This will only frustrate you if you're trying to lose weight! That's why the keto diet provides you with a healthy, filling diet and encourages you to exercise to spur on weight loss.

As we all know, eating too many carbohydrates is also correlated with a risk of developing type 2 diabetes. When your blood sugar levels rise, the body uses insulin to convert glucose into storage molecules and move it throughout the body. But if you are constantly having high blood sugar due to high carb intake, the body's insulin production system can

7

actually stop working. Your pancreas will continue to make insulin to keep up with the high blood sugar levels, but it cannot make enough or keep up with the demand. This is called insulin resistance. Having high blood sugar levels is called hyperglycemia and can lead to a risk of type 2 diabetes. Type 2 diabetes is the most common form of diabetes and can come with the risk of many other health symptoms.

Along with a risk of type 2 diabetes, eating too many carbohydrates can also increase your cholesterol numbers. Cholesterol is composed of three components: LDL cholesterol or the "bad" cholesterol, HDL or the "good" cholesterol, and a triglycerides number. Triglycerides are unhealthy fats that come from the food we consume. Alcohol, sugar, and excess calories in the body are converted into triglycerides which are stored in fat cells along the body. A high triglycerides count is linked to a high rate of heart disease. These fatty acids can build up in your arteries and increase your risk of blood clots, plaque buildup, and heart attack. When you are eating too many carbohydrates, the body stores excess carbs as triglycerides in the blood. Often, foods that are high in carbohydrates are also high in fat which means your arteries thicken due to unhealthy fat intake. The triglycerides can cause blockages in your blood flow which means your chances for a stroke or heart attack increase. If your triglyceride count increases due to high sugar intake, the HDL "good" cholesterol in your cholesterol makeup can actually decrease. As we see, too high a carbohydrate intake can wreak havoc on your cholesterol which can lead to cardiovascular disease.

There are so many other side effects of glucose and too much sugar that we often forget about them! Remember, glucose is a type of simple sugar so the body reacts as such when there's an influx of it in our bloodstream. When there's an unstable amount of sugar in our bloodstreams due to constant snacking on sweet treats, you can end up having mood swings or headaches as your body struggles to adjust. You may even feel false hunger pangs which causes you to overeat and gain weight. Often, people who binge on carbohydrates overeat because they feel they are not full enough despite intaking extra calories. With the additional sugar in your bloodstream, your body releases a rush of cortisol, the stress hormone, to try and stabilize your blood sugar levels. This sudden influx of hormones can cause a person to feel mood swings, irritable, and anxious as their body struggles to regulate itself.

Natural sugars such as those found in fruit tend to play little less of a role in increasing our blood sugar than high-fructose, highly processed sugary snacks. High-fructose corn syrup is cheaply produced and highly processed which is why it is used so often by beverage and snack companies. It's actually more than 20% sweeter than granulated sugar! This makes it a dangerous part of the diet for young kids and teenagers who are in puberty and need a healthy diet full of vitamins and minerals. In fact, a study by the Department of Agriculture found that people had lower levels of calcium, vitamins A, B-12, and C in their body when they tended to eat more sugar. The unnecessary amount of carbohydrates and sugar in your diet is depriving you of the opportunity for a healthy diet full of substances your body actually needs.

When your body realizes there's a sudden decrease in your carbohydrate intake, it begins the process of ketosis to create ketones for fuel. These tend to be more energy efficient than glucose molecules, which are produced as simple sugars from carbohydrates. Ketones are also metabolized faster than glucose and can bypass the glycolytic pathway. This gives you an instant boost of energy which you can sustain for longer than glucose could provide. Ketone molecules can even signal to the hypothalamus regarding energy levels and how fast glucose metabolism is occurring. That way, they can provide energy at a faster rate and regulate levels when necessary.

Chapter 2: Is the Keto Diet Right For You?

The keto diet can benefit many types of people, especially those who are obese or struggling to get rid of stubborn weight they can't shed. The diet has actually been used for nearly a century to treat seizures. Dating back to the 1920s, doctors believed that this form of modifying diet and greatly reducing carbohydrates would be effective to epileptic patients. Studies have shown that keto can reduce the risk of seizures, but since then, it's been used for its amazing weight loss abilities.

There are certain types of people who would greatly improve their health and benefit from following the keto diet. They include:

- Obese or overweight: People in this category can find this diet could help them get rid of weight they haven't been able to.
- People who have cancer: Studies have shown the ketogenic diet can help cancer patients.
- Chronic pain
- People at risk of neurodegenerative conditions such as Alzheimer's, Parkinson's, or dementia
- Women with PCOS
- People looking to gain more energy
- People looking to improve their mental and physical performance
- Athletes in low-endurance sports

No one diet can provide a cure to everyone's ailments, and there are certain people who should abstain from the keto diet due to their health. There are other methods for them to lose weight and become healthy instead of a regimented low-carbohydrate lifestyle that could be detrimental to them.

Keep in mind that no matter what your medical condition is, you should always consult a doctor first you to decide if the keto would be beneficial for you. If you have severe diabetes, this diet may not be able to help you and may interfere with your diabetes medication. People with severe health conditions or those on daily medication need to speak to their physician before making any changes to their diet.

Who are some other people who the keto diet may not be appropriate for? They include:

- Pregnant and breastfeeding women: Women in this condition will need extra calories to provide for their child, so they should not be dieting in any case.
- Children and teenagers: Young people going through puberty need to be eating healthy.
- High-endurance athletes: The keto diet may hinder some high-endurance athletes who require carbohydrates for their training.
- People with thyroid problems
- People with severe cases of diabetes
- People with adrenal fatigue conditions

Types of Keto Diets

This can come as a surprise, but there is more than one type of keto diet. There are four common approaches, and the other three are tweaked from the standard ketogenic diet that most people have heard of. All of them can still help you burn fat and lose weight but their method and macronutrient breakdown can vary. It's important to note that most of the research conducted regarding the keto diet is done using the standard diet, not the others. Unless a research study specifically states the subjects followed a different keto diet, participants would have been following the standard diet with minimal carbohydrate intake.

Here are the types of keto diets to understand how they differ from each other and what type of people they would work best for:

Standard Ketogenic Diet: This is the most common version that people follow and is great for beginners who simply want to lose weight and gain any potential health benefits. Most of the research and articles you read on the keto diet refers to this standard diet.

- This diet follows a breakdown as such: 75% calories from fat, 25% calories from protein, ~5% calories from carbohydrates. This should be from 20-50 grams of net carbs per day.

High-Protein Keto Diet: This diet is very similar to the standard keto diet but increases the protein intake. This is a targeted keto diet for those who are concerned about the lack of protein impairing muscle formation. Bodybuilders and weightlifters who are still interested in gaining the health benefits of keto but require extra protein for their activities could follow this diet.

Many people think that if you eat too much protein, it could push your body out of ketosis, but that's not true as long as you still limit your intake of carbohydrates which is key to following keto.

- This diet follows a breakdown as such: 60% calories from fat, 35% calories from protein, ~5% calories from carbohydrates.

Cyclical Ketogenic Diet (CKD): The cyclical keto diet follows a pattern of "on" and "off" days of eating a low-carbohydrate intake. You may follow keto for several days, then have a day or two where you consume a high amount of carbohydrates. The high carbohydrate phase can be anywhere from 24 to 48 hours and your carbohydrate intake would be nearly 70% of your caloric intake. This type of cyclical diet routine appeals to athletes and bodybuilders who are trying to maintain their body mass while still shedding extra fat.

The breakdown for this cyclical diet would be as follows:

- Standard ketogenic diet days (~5 days): 70-75% calories from fat, 20-25% calories from protein, ~5% calories from carbohydrates.
- Carbohydrate loading days (~2 days): 70% calories from carbohydrates, 20-25% calories from protein, 5-10% calories from fat.

Targeted Ketogenic Diet (TKD): This diet is one that schedules your carbohydrate intake to maximize your exercise performance. This fuels your muscles with instant glycogen during exercise to give you that last burst of energy to complete your workout.

People on this diet try and fit anywhere from 25-50 grams of carbohydrates about 30 minutes before their workout. High-glycemic carbohydrates like fructose and galactose should be avoided because they go to your liver, not your muscles, and end up converting into fatty lipids. This includes things like fresh fruit or fruit juices. Glucose and dextrose sugar supplies are the best things to eat to give your muscles a boost of energy. A substitute for carbohydrates for athletes could be to use MCT (medium chain triglycerides) oil which can help boost ketone levels. This is a great way to add to your daily fat intake and give you a boost of energy right before your workout.

It is important to note that most of the research regarding the keto diet is focused on the standard keto diet with the most minimum amount of carbohydrates. Targeted keto diets have commonly been used for athletes and bodybuilders who still want to gain the benefits of keto and lose weight, but need that burst of carbohydrates for training and exercise. The majority of scientific data though has been focused on the standard diet and how that impacts health. When we mention health benefits in the upcoming chapter, keep in mind that we are referring to the standard keto diet that the majority of the research is on.

Chapter 3: The Benefits and Drawbacks of the Keto Diet

There are many benefits of the keto diet that we can go over to convince you to give it a shot. Not only will you lose weight which might be people's initial goal, but you can improve your overall health and even protect yourself from future illnesses. We've listed some of the common benefits you may already know, and others you may not have been aware of. There may be some drawbacks to keto as well, but the benefits you gain far outweigh the hard parts of adjusting.

Benefits of the Keto Diet

Fat burning which results in weight loss. We have gone into detail about why exactly the keto diet can allow you to get rid of excess fat and how decreasing the amount of carbohydrates in your diet is directly related to fat-burning. The reason the diet has become such a popular sensation is because of the weight loss results it has produced! People have been able to follow this diet and still have their hunger sated, but lose weight at the same time! Studies have shown the keto diet can suppress your appetite and reduce your need for frequent snacking. Because you are eating less carbohydrates, your blood sugar levels are not going to be spiking as much, which means you will feel hungry less often. All these from training your body to use a different pathway to harness energy! There are two main categories of fat: the fat that is under your skin as a warmth layer, and visceral fat which accumulates at the abdomen. Visceral fat is most commonly what you will see in obese and overweight people. This fat can even spread around the organs which can cause inflammation. Low-carb diets are very effective at significantly reducing visceral fat quantities which is better for overall health. You've changed the type of diet you're eating, but you are in no way depriving yourself. If you couple this with frequent exercise throughout your week, you could lose weight even faster!

Stabilizes blood sugar levels and decreases risk for type 2 diabetes. For people who cannot keep their blood sugar stable or who suffer from diabetes but find themselves frequently snacking, the keto diet is a great way to stabilize your blood sugar levels. This diet has the majority of calories coming from fats and proteins, not carbohydrates which tend to cause blood sugar spikes. This means the body will produce less insulin to get rid of excess glucose. A study at the University of Padova in Padova, Italy followed obese and diabetic patients following the keto diet for a time span of 12 months. After a year, it was found that the patients following the keto diet had lost significantly more weight and reduced their fasting glucose levels. These are signs of reduced risk of diabetes. This diet is a great way for at-risk patients or patients who have a family history to stabilize their blood sugar levels and hopefully delay the onset of type 2 diabetes.

Improve many cardiovascular symptoms like reducing triglyceride fat, increasing HDL "good" cholesterol levels, and lowering blood pressure. It might seem to people that having a diet so high in fats will increase your risk of heart disease. But the keto diet proves that assumption wrong! You have changed your diet to accommodate healthy and high-quality fats which means you can reverse many symptoms of heart disease. These healthy fats boost your HDL "good" cholesterol level if that number has been low due to an unhealthy diet. If you've avoided fats in the past, the keto diet changes that and boosts your good cholesterol number. It also decreases the amount of triglyceride fatty acids in your bloodstream. A high amount of triglycerides in the blood can lead to increased risk of heart disease. High carbohydrate consumption tends to increase triglyceride count in the blood. When people follow a diet like a keto diet where they drastically reduce their carbs, they can successfully decrease their triglyceride fatty acid count. Hypertension, or high blood pressure, is also linked with stroke and heart disease. Low-carb diets have proven very effective in reducing blood pressure. A study found that compared to other diet groups tested, the group participating in a low-carb diet lowered their systolic blood pressure by almost 8 mm HG—that is two times as much as the other groups! In fact, a 2018 study on cardiovascular health found that the keto diet can improve as many 22 out of 26 risk factors! Decreasing these risk factors is a great way to prevent the onset of any disease of the heart or blood vessels, especially if you are battling a family history.

Decrease inflammation in the body. A 2015 research study at the Yale School of Medicine found that the ketogenic diet is significantly helpful in reducing inflammation and can reduce the risk of the other health problems associated with inflammation. Inflammation is linked with many minor and severe health condition such as eczema, acne, autoimmune conditions, psoriasis, arthritis, and irritable bowel syndrome. The research found that the keto diet successfully produces BHB, a ketone that inhibits an inflammatory response in the body. Another 2008 research study in The New England Journal of Medicine found that participants on the keto diet had a reduced amount of C-reactive proteins (hsCRPs) in their blood. This is a marker linked to high inflammation in the body. The keto diet followers had nearly 40% less hsCRPs in their blood count! By following a low-carb diet which allows the body to more regularly produce ketones by way of ketosis, you could prevent inflammation from occurring.

Have higher energy levels and a better night's sleep. Though you may initially feel sluggish for a few days after you make the switch to the keto diet, the research proves that being on keto will actually increase your energy levels. That's because the body is now using a more rich source of energy— fat, instead of the "quick" source of carbohydrates. Ketones provide a longer lasting source of energy than glucose molecules. Participants found that once they made it through the adjustment phase of the "keto flu", they felt more energized and energetic than they had before. Along with increased energy throughout the day, the keto diet provides a better night's sleep by decreasing the REM (rapid eye movement) cycle. There's no exact research on the phenomenon, but it could be that the brain expends more energy producing ketones which then allows the body to rest better at night. That means better quality and less interrupted sleep.

Improves mental clarity. When the body follows a diet loaded on carbohydrates, the brain uses glucose energy for all its functioning. But research has shown that ketones are a more rich energy source for brain function than glucose molecules. When following a low-carb diet, the brain has drastically reduced carbohydrate intake and has nearly 75% of calories coming from high-quality fats. Neurologists believe that it means the neurons and brain mitochondria have a more stable and sustained energy source to function at their highest level. Many research studies have found that patients on the keto diet have better memory recall, higher cognitive functioning, and less susceptible to phases of dementia. Along with less frequent migraines and increased attention to detail, it's easy to see why people feel the keto diet allows them to function at their top mental clarity level.

Can reduce the risk of cancer. This can sound like a bit of a stretch, but the keto diet has been studied extensively to see how it can treat certain types of cancers in patients. Many researchers have theorized that cancer cells use insulin receptors to attract glucose and use that as fuel to multiply and survive in the body. That means cancer continues to spread despite a person trying to eat healthily. When following the keto diet, cancer patients are reducing their carbohydrate intake and allowing their body to use ketosis to harness energy from ketones. This reduces glucose in the body and, hopefully, cancer cells cannot flourish and replicate.

Decrease the side effects of neurodegenerative diseases like Alzheimer's, epilepsy, and Parkinson's disease. Experiments on the keto diet have found that energy from ketones in the body is correlated with greater memory recall and higher cognitive functioning. Ketones can preserve a high level of functioning in brain cells and prevent injury or loss of neural cells. This can reduce the risk of neurodegenerative diseases as we mentioned above. In fact, the keto diet was created in the 1920s to treat epilepsy in children. Many studies have found that patients with conditions like Parkinson's and Alzheimer's were able to improve their mental condition when following a low-carb diet. This could be because you're restricting the body's intake of sugar which minimizes any potential blood sugar spikes that the body's neuron cells have to adjust to.

Can regulate hormone levels in women with PCOS (polycystic ovary syndrome) and PMS (pre-menstrual syndrome). PCOS is a condition that can cause infertility in more than 50% of the women who suffer from it. It can be a heartbreaking condition for young couples who are trying to conceive a child. There is no cure for this condition, but it's believed that it's caused by high insulin levels. High insulin levels in the body cause the ovaries to produce more sex-hormones which can lead to conditions like mood swings, fatigue, obesity, hair growth, acne, and infertility. The keto diet has been recommended to many women suffering from PCOS as a way to regulate their insulin and hormone levels. This regulation could reduce the hormones secreted by the body and increase their chances of getting pregnant. A 2005 study even resulted in two women following the keto diet conceiving a child! The keto diet is highly recommended to regulate hormone levels because hormone molecules are created from cholesterol, fat molecules, and amino acid proteins. That's exactly what the keto diet prescribes! With a high intake of quality proteins and fats, the body can create hormones to regulate any occurring imbalances. The keto diet can even regulate slight hormone imbalances that occur before a woman's menstrual cycle. PMS can cause things like mood swings, acne, and headaches at that time of the month, but by minimizing your sugar intake, you can regulate blood sugar levels for a more stable menstrual cycle.

Reduce how much stress hormone the body secretes. As we explained before, the body's blood sugar levels are constantly reacting to its carbohydrate intake. When you have something with carbs or sugar, your blood sugar spike and the body has to quickly stabilize those levels. When that happens, the body's hormonal system produces cortisol, which is known as the stress hormone. When the body secretes too much cortisol, it can result in symptoms like weight gain, dizziness, hunger pangs, mood swings, and headaches. This can be dangerous because it can lead to overeating even when the body isn't hungry, which is why stressed people often feel they've gained weight. Following the keto diet minimizes the body's carbohydrate intake drastically which means less blood sugar spikes and less need for cortisol to be secreted. This means the adrenal glands feel less stress and your glands can work normally to recognize stressful situations instead of being driven into action with every blood sugar spike.

Can reduce the feelings of depression. Studies have shown that rats on the ketogenic diet displayed less despair in their movements compared on the control diet group— they were more active and showed less signs of hopelessness. Such signs are what occurs when someone is suffering from depression. Movement is considered one of the most important anti-depressants out there. Think about when you've felt sad or depressed and can't seem to get off the couch! Instead, the keto diet allowed these test groups to feel more energetic which means they were less likely to be sedentary and be consumed by feelings of helplessness. This is especially key for people suffering from depression and who wish for energy to resume their normal routine. The keto diet also produces an anti-inflammatory effect on the brain which may, in the long run, improve brain function. This means it could potentially alter the neurochemical effects of depression that people struggle to combat.

Drawbacks of the Keto Diet

Counting calories can be tough to get used to.
Although the keto diet has changed millions of lives through weight loss and health benefits, the truth is, it can be a struggle for some beginners to get used to. Often, people are used to just trimming their portion size when on a diet or

avoiding what they can't eat so they aren't tempted. With the keto diet, you need to be a little more precise than that! Counting calories, net carbs, fat intake, and protein per serving is necessary to ensure you are feeling the keto diet breakdown. If your proportions are incorrect, it could mean you gain weight instead! This adaption period for beginners can be tough, especially if you have a habit of snacking between meals. But once you realize why this breakdown and calorie counting is so important, you may be more appreciative of the process. Having a breakdown is great to look back at in case you aren't losing weight as you expected. You can easily find free calorie counter apps that will have you input serving information and will track your daily intake.

Your brain may need some time to adjust. Despite the case we've made about the body adjusting to ketosis as an alternative pathway for energy, the truth is that your body and brain may feel the deprivation of carbohydrates before it adjusts. That means you feel slow and sluggish for the first week or so and might feel like you're not performing at your optimal mental alertness. Sometimes, people go through these initial rough days and give up; they feel this isn't what they signed up and that they're not seeing the weight loss results they were promised. You have to remember that your body is completely changing the way it harnesses energy from glucose to ketones. That adjustment takes some time for your body to now go through the process of ketosis. As long as you don't give up and power through it, you will see the benefits after! We will have some tips on how to battle the "keto flu" as it is coined in our next chapter.

Carbohydrates help your athletic performance. If you are an athlete or play high-endurance sports, you may be skeptical about the keto diet because a low-carb diet could result in poor performance. Though there are tweaked keto diets you can follow that allow for a greater amount of carbohydrates intake, the truth is that most athletes rely on carbohydrates for a quick burst of energy to work out. If you are playing high-endurance sports without a lot of breaks, like soccer or rugby, or you lift a large amount of weights for your workouts, the keto diet may not be for you. In fact, the International Olympic Committee has urged athletes to avoid low-carbohydrate diets because it can impact their performance and cause injury when training. Although there are still athletes who use this diet for the other health benefits such as more energy, weight loss, and mental clarity, it might not be the perfect diet for you depending on your athletic needs.

You may be craving carbohydrates! That old adage is true: you always want what you can't have! With the keto diet, you are drastically reducing your carbohydrate intake from what it was. For most people, carbs make up more than half their diet. To go from that to a measly 5% can be quite tough! You may find yourself craving your go-to carbohydrate snacks and tempted by what is around you. Keep in mind that this initial period of cravings will pass and the keto diet actually helps to suppress your appetite when you have successfully achieved the state of ketosis. That means you'll feel less hungry and need less snacks throughout meals. Try and avoid situations where you're tempted by carbs and keep yourself busy so you aren't reaching for what you shouldn't have. You can do it!

After going over the pros and cons of the keto diet, it's easy to see why the pros seem to win! This diet can help you get rid of stubborn weight you've gained, but also prevent and ease symptoms of many conditions you may have or be at risk of. The adjustment period can be a bit tough and you have to get used to counting calories and watching the breakdown of your calories, but many have felt once they have adjusted, this diet is worth it!

Chapter 4: The Side Effects of the Keto Diet

As we've mentioned previously, the keto diet isn't a magical remedy to help you get rid of stubborn weight and set you on a healthier lifestyle. It comes with its share of adjustments and a learning curve that beginners have to overcome. The research has shown that the keto diet proves successful in improving health, but it takes some steps to get there. Your body has to make the switch from using simple carbohydrates to create glucose for energy and now go through the ketosis process to use the energy-rich ketone molecules. Just as you have to train your body when you are quitting an addiction or getting into shape for a marathon, it takes some time to adjust, but you will feel better once you have!

What are some of the side effects of being on the keto diet? You might notice some of these symptoms show up after you've made the switch to keto and drastically reduced your carbohydrates intake. Your body will be adjusting and realizing that, with the harsh decrease in carbohydrates, it has to go through ketosis now to create fuel. You can purchase blood strips or urine strips that can positively test for signs your body is in ketosis, but many trainers find those inaccurate. Instead, they recommend monitoring your body and looking for key physical signs that will indicate your body's successful push into ketosis. We will go over some of these signs below and how you can combat them.

Increased Urination: As your body adjusts to ketosis, it begins to first get rid of excess water weight by eliminating excess minerals like sodium, magnesium, and potassium. A decrease in carbohydrate intake means the body will produce less insulin and secrete excess insulin through urination as well. This can mean extra trips to the bathroom! In fact, the body produces the ketone acetoacetate that can be excreted only through urination. But once your body adjusts to ketosis, your system will naturally adjust. Until then, it's important you continue to drink enough water and remain hydrated.

Bad Breath: The increased ketone levels in your body also produce a molecule called acetone. This is one of the molecules created during ketosis and some describe it as having a very potent distinct smell, like ripe fruit or nail polish remover. When mixed with saliva, this smell can become very strong and you'll notice you're suffering from bad breath. The good news is that it is temporary! This is a sign the ketosis is processing in your body and successfully burning fats for fuel. Many people report the smell will go away in a week or two as the body completely adapts to your new diet. Until then, here are some tips to help you fight the problem.

- Brush your teeth at least twice a day and practice good oral hygiene.
- Chew gum or have mints handy to try and mask the smell.
- Drink plenty of water. Bad breath can increase if you have less saliva from dry mouth.

Drowsiness or Dizziness: Due to the loss of water weight and losing minerals from the body, this can make you feel fatigued, lightheaded, drowsy and dizzy as your body adjusts. To counteract these effects, here are some things you can try:

- Eat foods rich in potassium such as broccoli, avocados, poultry, and dairy.
- Season your food with some extra salt when cooking or use regular sodium broth for soups and dishes. This increases your salt intake to help you regain electrolyte balance.
- You can also add an over the counter magnesium supplement to your routine before bed every night. But, it is important you consult your doctor before taking any oral supplements.

Low Blood Sugar: This is known as hypoglycemia which is very common when someone has started keto and the body is experiencing the sudden decrease in carbohydrates. When your diet had consisted of more than 50% carbohydrates, it's going to be hard to adjust to a sudden 5%—your body will feel the effects! You may be acquainted with short-term episodes of low blood sugar and may also feel shaky, hungry, or tired until your body begins to adjust. To combat this:

- Be sure you aren't going hungry for too long. If it's not mealtime, at least have a healthy keto-friendly snack.
- Begin your keto diet slowly if you are worried about the sudden decline in carbohydrates. Slowly cut back instead of going completely down to 5%.

Constipation or Diarrhea: When your diet has changed so drastically by going on keto, it's only natural that your body will go through some digestive issues as it adjusts. Constipation could occur because of the high protein and fat content you're suddenly eating. On the flip side, some people might experience diarrhea as they adjust to the higher fat intake and low-carbohydrate count. Here are some tips to help combat digestive issues:

- Be sure you're staying hydrated. Dehydration occurs as you lose fluids and will only worsen constipation.
- Eat a high intake of fibrous vegetables to get your digestive tract moving. If you feel you're not getting enough fiber through vegetables, include a fiber supplemental powder in your drinks or food to increase your intake.
- Some trainers would recommend cutting back on nut and dairy consumption which can cause digestive issues.

Muscle Cramps: These can occur when you first start keto and your body is getting rid of water weight and excess minerals. This can cause an electrolyte imbalance in your muscles which means you can feel muscle cramps, especially in your legs where the larger muscles are located. In order to deal with the side effects, you should:

- Stay hydrated to keep your muscles healthy. Make sure you're drinking enough water.
- Increase your salt intake to counteract the loss of minerals. You could also try drinking electrolyte drinks to ensure you're getting enough intake.
- A magnesium supplement can also help combat muscle cramps, but be sure you ask your doctor before adding any medication to your diet.

What Is the Keto Flu and How To Fight It

The most common side effect of keto is something that has been coined "the keto flu" by people who have experienced it. That's because the symptoms are very similar for flu-like symptoms you would suffer, including headaches, tiredness, confusion, dizziness, vomiting, stomach pain, poor focus, difficulty sleeping, drowsiness, nausea, and irritability. These symptoms can appear within the first 2-4 days of beginning the keto diet as your body struggles to adjust to the sudden decrease in carbohydrates.

To put it simply, it's like your body is in "withdrawal" from lack of carbohydrates. You're going from having carbohydrates be such a large part of the diet anywhere from 60-70%, to a drastic change of only around 5%. These flu symptoms can be minor or very severe depending on each person. It can depend on what your previous level of sugar and carb consumption was or if you already eat healthy meals. Genetics, your individual physical fitness, and electrolyte and water intake can all make an impact on how your body will adjust to the keto diet and how quickly it will get over the keto flu. If you had slowly decreased your carbohydrate intake before going on keto, you could adjust better. If you are one of those people who are sure to stay hydrated and take electrolytes, it could help you fight symptoms even more.

These keto flu symptoms can be disheartening to people who are enthusiastic about switching to keto and seeing quick results. This slump can feel exhausting when you're trying to follow a new diet plan and maybe even incorporate exercise into your routine to lose weight faster. But we urge you to stay motivated and not give up! These symptoms are a natural reaction of your body as it adjusts to the new diet and pushes itself into ketosis. These symptoms are temporary and will pass. After they do, you'll have more energy and more focus to adjust to your new lifestyle.

Here are some tips you can follow to beat the keto flu.

Be sure you're staying hydrated. We've mentioned this again and again because it's so important! Staying hydrated is critical for every individual, but when you're following the keto diet, it's very important you have enough water intake. The ketosis process starts with causing you to shed water weight. That means frequent urination and loss of water. Glycogen levels also decrease as water leaves the body. That means you have more cause to feel dizzy, lightheaded, and tired. To combat these symptoms, you should ensure you're drinking enough water to replenish your body and protect sensitive issues. The Mayo Clinic recommends at least 15 cups a day for men and 11-12 cups per day for women. This can sound like a lot, so a great tip is to have a reusable water bottle that you can fill throughout the day. Infusing your water with low-calorie fruit or mint leaves is a great way to put a small amount of flavor without adding empty calories.

Get enough electrolytes and salt in your diet. With less frequent blood sugar spikes due to a low intake of carbohydrates, the body has to release excess insulin in the body. That happens via the kidneys which release sodium through frequent urination. Your body is getting rid of excess minerals like magnesium, sodium, and potassium, which means that you have to do something to combat the electrolyte imbalance in our body. If your body's levels become too low, that can result in those flu-like symptoms we mentioned above like drowsiness, nausea, tiredness, and muscle cramps. To keep your body supplied with electrolytes, be sure you're using iodized salt in your cooking and seasoning of food. Some keto researchers recommend an extra 1-2 teaspoons of table salt when on the keto diet to correct any electrolyte imbalance. Himalayan salt can be a great addition to your meals and spice cabinet as well. Just a pinch of it contains more than 80 minerals! Bone broth is also considered a great dish that is hydrating and high in electrolytes. It's also important to incorporate more foods into your diet that are rich in electrolytes. This will ensure you're getting the minerals you need and preventing flu-like symptoms due to electrolyte imbalance. Here are some of the examples of the foods you can include in your diet:

- Magnesium: almonds, quinoa, cashews, avocado, spinach
- Sodium: iodized table salt, Himalayan salt, bone broth
- Potassium: spinach, broccoli, mushrooms, dates

Don't be ashamed to start slow. If you're worried about the adjustment to keto and suffering from the keto flu for a few weeks which could interfere with your daily life, it is completely okay to take a step back and ease yourself into keto. Slashing those carbohydrates so drastically can be tough! There's no shame in slowly decreasing your carbohydrate intake over a week or two. If you know it will be an adjustment and your diet is loaded with sugars and carbs, then take some time to slowly ease back in your diet one meal and one snack at a time. Or you can start by following a cyclical keto diet which means a few days "on" keto and a few days off. This will allow you to feel more confident as you begin keto and feel more comfortable with the reduced amount of carbohydrates.

Avoid high-endurance exercise. If you're an athlete or if you schedule workouts at the gym throughout the week, when you're suffering from the keto flu, it might be a good idea to avoid stressful exercise. It could actually cause injury because you will be feeling tired and weak and you will be experiencing muscle cramps or pain. That means you could injure yourself when participating in high-endurance exercises or lifting heavy weights. Sit out on the Cross Fit, heavy weightlifting, and intense aerobic workouts that you may not have the energy for. Once you feel better and have gotten over the keto flu "hump," you can return to your exercise routine and feel more energetic than ever. Be sure to give your body the time it needs to adjust and not push it too hard.

Try light exercises like yoga or Pilates. As we mentioned above, you should skip any high-endurance workout routines, but some light exercise could help you feel better as you adjust to the keto diet. These include more relaxing exercises like yoga, Pilates, or just a walk around the block after dinner. This will help you mentally, help any digestive issues, and push your body to keep burning fat and enter the state of ketosis. This activity depends on your physical health, of course. If you're feeling lightheaded or dizzy due to the keto flu, then you should abstain from physical activity that could worsen your symptoms. Otherwise, breathing exercises, stretching, and yoga are great ways to relax your body and stay active without the high-intensity workout.

Keep track of your macros. This is why it's so important when beginning the keto diet to ensure you're keeping track of what you're eating and your caloric breakdown. If you're not eating enough high-quality fat, then your body will not be able to push itself towards ketosis. If your carbohydrate breakdown is higher than it needs to be, then your body will continue to rely on glucose. Having a breakdown of what you're eating, including snacks throughout the day, will help you have an idea of your macro breakdown and what you need to change if you're still not feeling the benefits of keto a few weeks down the line.

Get a good night's sleep. This can be tough advice if one of your symptoms of the keto flu is having difficulty sleeping. But the more you can rest and recharge your body, the more refreshed you will feel the next day. This will fight the tiredness you are feeling as your body adjusts to the new diet. Sleeping also decreases the amount of stress hormones being secreted by the body. Here are some tips to help you get a good night's rest:

- Avoid caffeine in the evenings before bedtime
- Stay off screens and stop working about an hour before bed and spend some time relaxing
- Meditating, breathing exercises, or prayer may help you clear your mind and get rid of stressful thoughts
- Take a magnesium or melatonin supplement to help your body get to sleep faster (be sure you speak to a doctor before taking any over the counter medication!)

Increase your carbohydrates count, if necessary. If you still feel like you're battling the keto flu weeks after you've made the switch to a keto diet, you can try adding some additional healthy carb to your diet. This might ease your symptoms. It will not be following the standard keto diet as your carbohydrates count will be too high, but it gives your body more time to adjust and could fight back on those symptoms that are making you feel sluggish and slow. Try adding "clean" carbohydrates like berries, vegetables, or seeds. If this helps ease your symptoms, then slowly decrease your carbohydrates amount so you are back on the keto level of around 5%. Remember, unless you are having the minimum amount of carbohydrates, your body will not go into the stage of ketosis. That's when the maximum weight loss and health benefits will occur.

Include some ketone supplements. These supplements are a healthy way to push your body towards ketosis. They give your body some extra ketones which will give you energy when you are struggling with the keto flu. Even just a spoonful of ketone powder in your morning smoothie may make the difference if you are still fighting the keto flu and looking for that burst of energy from ketosis. MCT oil is also a great addition to your diet. It's made of high-quality fat triglycerides that the body can naturally use to make energy. These fats are harnessed by the liver to create ketones. Many beginners on the keto diet will use MCT oil as a way to give their body an extra burst of energy as they're waiting for their body to naturally go into ketosis.

Be patient! These symptoms of keto flu can make you feel disappointed that you aren't seeing those amazing benefits of keto that we've talked about—or that you're not losing weight despite your complete change in diet. These symptoms are to be expected because you are changing how your body is now going to harness energy. After having a diet filled with mostly carbohydrates, your body is now going to push itself to use the fat it has stored for energy. These "keto flu" symptoms will go away once your body adjusts and you'll be able to recognize other physical symptoms that you are now in ketosis. With that burst of energy, mental clarity, and weight loss, you'll be more motivated to follow the keto diet and include exercise in your routine. Until then, be patient with your body as you start this new lifestyle and remind yourself that an adjustment process is common with all lifestyle changes.

Chapter 5: What You Can and Cannot Eat on Keto?

When starting a new diet, it's important to know exactly what you can and cannot eat. When you think of dieting, you might think of nothing but agonizing salads and low-fat foods that offer little flavor options. With the keto diet, it might surprise you how many foods you are allowed to eat in comparison to what you can't! In fact, there's such a richness in foods you can eat that you will hardly believe you're following a diet lifestyle! Remember, it's all about keeping track of your macro intake so your carbohydrates stay slow. 75% fat, 20% protein, ~5% carbohydrates. This means you can have a lowly carbohydrate intake but you want to be sure you're counting net carbs so it only accounts for 5% of your total. The closer you follow this standard keto diet breakdown, the more weight loss results you will see.

Foods You Can Eat

Meat: If you're a meat-lover, then the keto diet is perfect for you! Your usual sources of protein are allowed and recommended on keto. It is encouraged that you have a variety of protein sources to get the vitamins and minerals you need. You want to keep in mind that the keto diet's breakdown is not the largest amount of protein—it's fat. So you don't need a huge intake of meat, but it can be a great source of fuel throughout your day. When choosing your meat cuts, try choosing fattier cuts like a ribeye steak. That way, you're also adding to your fat intake for the day. If you're eating too much protein, that will actually get converted into glucose and slow your body's progress to ketosis. This is why monitoring your macros is so important, to ensure you're properly following the recommended keto scale. It is encouraged on keto that you try and buy organic and grass-fed cuts of meat. This can be a little pricier, but researchers believe it's healthier because it's less risk of ingesting any hormones or pesticides from the animal. Keto is all about eating high-quality foods to achieve the results you want. You also want to avoid processed meats like cold cuts or sausages which might contain hidden carbs. Meat sources include:

- Poultry: chicken, turkey
- Goat meat
- Lamb meat
- Beef: ground beef, roasts, steak
- Organ meats
- Pork: bacon, ham, pork chops, pork loin

Fish and Seafood: Fish is another essential protein source and is rich in omega-3 fatty acids. This is important for the brain and vision health and keeps your heart healthy by increasing good cholesterol and decreasing blood pressure. If you're already an avid seafood lover, this is great news. If you aren't, try a variety of fish and find a favorite that you may prefer. There are many types available in local grocery stores or at specialized fish stores. Catfish, flounder, mahi-mahi, halibut, salmon, tilapia, tuna—don't stop at just one type! Seafood also includes other protein sources like lobster, mussels, shrimp, oysters, and clams.

Eggs: Eggs are another great source of protein and can make for a great snack. Scrambled, fried, or boiled—they are a great addition to a meal as a side to increase your protein intake and gain healthy fats. Try and buy free-range eggs as much as you can so you feel secure they are hormone-free.

Dairy: Dairy is also a common part of the keto diet though you want to stay away from products that have a great amount of carbohydrates. If you're consuming too much dairy that is loaded with carbs, you may unknowingly be increasing your carbohydrate intake which means your body will not be in ketosis. Some dairy products are also rich in protein, so it's important you keep that in mind when pairing dairy with a protein dish. Also, be sure you are choosing raw or organic dairy products that are full-fat dairy instead of a low-fat or fat-free option. This will allow you to increase your fat intake and feel full longer. The most common dairy products consumed on keto are cheeses, heavy cream, and ghee or butter used for frying. Ghee is clarified butter often used in Asia. It has a more nutty flavor that can add taste to your food. Cream cheese, mayonnaise, and Greek yogurt are also great to use for spreads. You want to try and avoid condensed or evaporated milk because they are very high in sugar. Almond milk is a great alternative and is delicious for making keto-friendly smoothies. Be sure you're choosing the unsweetened version of almond milk so you aren't getting extra carbs through sugar. Dairy sources include:

- Half-and-half, heavy cream (in tea or coffee)
- Hard cheeses (swiss, cheddar, feta, Parmesan)
- Soft cheeses (brie, colby, mozzarella)
- Cream cheese, cottage cheese, sour cream
- Full-fat Greek yogurt
- Mayonnaise

Vegetables: With vegetables and fruits, you are allowed to have a diet with a rich variety of them, but it's important you're aware of the net carbohydrates intake you would be consuming. Again, it's all about maintaining that low-carbohydrate intake level so your body can follow the route to ketosis. Vegetables that grow underground are higher in carbohydrates, such as potatoes, corn, peas, yams, beans, and sweet potatoes. Avoid starchy vegetables. Colorful vegetables like eggplant, peppers, and tomatoes are actually high in carbohydrates. Other vegetables are ones you can eat in moderation, but again, be aware of your carbohydrate intake. Lettuce, celery, cauliflower, mushrooms, and broccoli are packed with vitamins and minerals but still low in carbohydrates. Leafy green vegetables are also keto-friendly and great as a base for salads.

Here is some important nutritional information regarding commonly consumed vegetables on the keto diet:

1 cup	Net Carbs
Celery	1.39 grams
Asparagus	1.8 grams
Spinach	1.48 grams
Bell Pepper	2.9 grams
Cauliflower	2.98 grams
Cucumber	3.18 grams
Broccoli	4 grams
Kale	5.25 grams
Turnips	4.65 grams
Brussel Sprouts	5.13 grams
Carrots	6.79 grams
Onions	7.64 grams

Fruit: This category can be a little tricky on keto simply because so many fruits are high in natural sugars and carbohydrates. Though fruits are very healthy, it's important that you're aware of which should be included on the keto diet and which shouldn't. For example, just 6 ounces of raspberries contains almost 88 calories and 10 grams of carbohydrates! One banana can have up to 25 grams of net carbs! So you can see how having too much fruit could skew your keto macro count and inadvertently increase your carbohydrate intake. There are some fruits that have a low-carbohydrate count that you can include in your diet such as avocados, blackberries, or clementines. You want to try and reach for the "less" naturally sweet fruits in each category. Blackberries are less sweet than strawberries and raspberries, and clementines tend to be less sweet than grapefruits or oranges. Olives are low in carbs and are a great source of fat, too! They can be a great fat content to add to your salad.

Here is some important nutritional information regarding commonly consumed fruit on the keto diet:

1 cup	Net Carbs
Avocado	2.7 grams
Lemon	6 carbs
Cantaloupe	8.3 grams
Strawberries	8.8 grams

Clementine	7.8 grams
Raspberries	6.8 grams
Kiwi	9 grams
Blackberries	6.4 grams
Pear	8 grams
Grapes	26 grams
Orange	27 grams
Pineapple	20 grams

Nuts and Seeds: Raw nuts are a great way to add flavor and texture to your meal. They can work as a snack, but you want to be sure you are avoiding high-carb nuts. Remember, snacking, in general, will increase your blood sugar and may slow your weight loss progress. You also want to be sure you're not having too many nuts because they are often high in protein and omega-6 fatty acids as well. Make sure your nuts are in the raw form and are not candied or salted because those are unnecessary calories that are not healthy.

- Low-carbohydrate nuts: brazil nuts, pecans, macadamia nuts
- Moderate-carbohydrate nuts: almonds, hazelnuts, pine nuts, walnuts
- High-carbohydrate nuts: cashews, pistachios

Drinks: We've spoken many times of the importance of water on the keto diet. Considering that your body is two-thirds water, it's important that you are staying hydrated, especially when first adjusting to keto and fighting off any transitional symptoms. Researchers recommend drinking at least 1 gallon of water daily on keto, if possible! Try adding some infused ice cubes with mint leaves or keto-friendly fruit to add more flavor to your water. The more you drink, the better it will be for your system. The keto diet has a diuretic side effect which means you will be urinating more to get rid of excess water weight, so you need to be replenishing fluids as well. You can have keto-friendly tea or coffee as well and increase your fat content by adding heavy whipping cream. But too much caffeine will stop your weight loss, so you should try and limit it to 2 cups a day. And make sure you're not using sugar in your beverages! That's empty calories you don't need! Some great sources of hydration include:

- Water: This will be your most reached for source of hydration. Sparkling water is a great alternative, but be sure you check that there's no carbohydrates.
- Coffee: Make sure it's keto-friendly and that you aren't using sugar or high-carb creamers. Coffee has the

added benefit of making you feel more full than you are so it can prevent you from excess snacking.

- Tea: Stick with black or green tea which has health benefits.
- Almond or coconut milk: Be sure you're using the unsweetened version!
- Alcohol: Alcohol is allowed in moderation, though hard liquor tends to be lower in calories compared to beer or wine.
- Bone broth: This dish is full of vitamins and minerals, and is very hydrating too!

Sauces and Condiments: This can be a little bit of a gray area on keto simply because there can be many added sugar in just a dollop of sauce. That's why, it's very important to always check the nutrition label to ensure you're not going over in carbs when adding a little bit of condiment to your dish. If you want to be safe, then it's best just to avoid all pre-made sauces and condiments to ensure you're not getting any unnecessary sugars and artificial sweeteners. But if you're one of those people who is used to sauces or gravies on your food, it's important that you read the label before adding it to your food. Try and see if there's any low-carb options in your grocery store. Condiments that tend to be fine for the keto diet include:

- Ketchup (low or no sugar)
- Mustard
- Mayonnaise (choose cage-free when you can)
- Horseradish
- Relish (low or no sugar)
- Salad dressings (choose fattier dressings like Caesar or ranch and unsweetened vinaigrettes)
- Hot sauce
- Worcestershire sauce

The key thing to remember is to keep your condiment usage on the safe side and use them moderately over the week. You may ruin a healthy low-carb meal if you add too much to your dish!

Foods to Avoid

Whole Grains and Starches: Typically, we know that whole grains are much healthier for us than refined bread, but on the keto diet, you still want to stay away from simple sugars and carbohydrates. That includes things like cereal, rice, corn, quinoa, pasta, and whole wheat bread so you can keep your carbohydrate count low. Beans and lentils are also high in carbohydrates and should be avoided.

Sugars: Of course, you want to stay away from sugars such as sweets, candy, cakes, cookies, fruit drinks, and soda. Even "vitamin water" tends to be high in sugar. We recommend staying away from sugar-free treats like candy or ice cream as well because they tend to be high in artificial sweeteners that still spike your blood sugar. Be sure you're reading the label when trying a new food to make sure you're not getting any hidden sugars. Try and limit artificial sweeteners as well, though they can be used in moderation to add some sweetness to smoothies or keto-friendly snacks. Diet soda should also be cut out of your diet because of the artificial sweeteners in it.

Root Vegetables: As we mentioned above, you want to stay from root vegetables that tend to be high in nutrients because they grow underneath the soil. That means things like carrots, turnips, potatoes, sweet potatoes, ginger, yams, beets, and turnips. Instead, try and find those low-carb vegetables that can be filling and still be a healthy addition to your meals. Leafy green vegetables like broccoli and kale are also great for salads or sautéed as a side.

Fruits High in Sugar: As we mentioned above, you have to be careful with fruits because even just a cup of fruit for a healthy snack can fill your daily carbohydrate count! Focus on low-carb fruits such as avocados, honeydew, watermelon, cucumbers and peaches which are still filling and can satisfy your sugar craving.

Margarine, Trans Fats, and Some Oils: Margarine is an unhealthy substitute for butter that many people aren't aware of. It has no health benefits and doesn't have the delicious, filling taste that butter or ghee does when it comes to cooking. The high omega-6 content in it makes it an ingredient you should stay away from. Trans fats are linked to a high risk of cardiovascular disease as well. Instead of oils like sunflower or canola oil that can be unhealthy for you, try using oils with higher fat contents like avocado oil or ghee. This increases your fat intake for whatever you're cooking so you meet your daily macro limit.

Low-Fat Foods: It's the opposite of what you may be advised on other diets. But with keto, you want to reach for the full-fat option instead of low or moderate fat. Your daily fat content should be around 75% of your daily caloric intake so it's important that you are being sure to include those calories even in the little things like yogurt, cuts of meat, oil, and salad dressings.

Chapter 6: Starting and Maintaining a Keto Diet

How to Get Started on Keto

First, clean out your kitchen. You want to get rid of anything that is high in carbohydrates and the things that you know you cannot consume on keto. That means sodas, bread, pasta, candy, and processed snacks. The more strictly you want to follow your keto routine, the more you need to remove temptation from your diet.

Be aware of your sugar and carb intake. This is a good time to be aware of how much sugar you consume without knowing. Whether it's a quick snack or a teaspoon of sugar in your coffee, it's important you are cognizant so you can slowly cut back on this.

Look up recipes and meal plan. Meal plans are a great way to prepare meals ahead of time. That means you're more likely to follow keto instead of trying to find an alternative. Look up meals that you can make given your cooking level and how much time you have.

Put together a grocery list of keto-friendly items. Going by the last chapter where we listed what you should include on your new keto grocery list, pick out things that you like to eat and that you can plan your meals around. Be sure you're including sources of protein, vegetables, and snacks.

Incorporate a variety of protein and vegetables in your diet. By now, you should have an understanding of what is "allowed" on keto and what isn't. That means you should try and have a variety of protein sources and vegetables on your shopping list. This way you won't get bored with your diet and have new flavors and dishes to try. If you're not already a veggie lover, try new vegetables to see how you like them, and expand your palette to include fish and seafood if you've always leaned more toward meat.

Buy keto-friendly snacks. Whether that's a cheese platter, veggie sticks, or nuts and seeds, it's important you have a healthy snack to reach for so you don't break your diet. The last thing you want to do is end a good keto day with an unhealthy carbohydrate-loaded snack. Look up keto snack recipes like fat bombs or smoothies and be sure you have those ingredients stocked.

Have appropriate measuring cups or a food scale. This will prevent you from overeating and allow you to properly measure ingredients when trying a new recipe. Properly portioning your food will be very important and allow you to make the correct amount of servings so you can eat one and store the rest as part of the meal plan prep.

Count your calories. Don't forget that hidden carbs count! Keep track of your carbs throughout the day so you are aware of how much you are eating daily and what percent of your intake is from fat, protein, and carbohydrates.

Don't stress! The more stressed you are, the more likely your body is to produce false hunger signals which can result in overeating. If you are stressed and worried about the keto diet, then that's not resulting in your blood sugar levels being stable. Embark it as a new and positive change in your life! Take the time every day to relax and be motivated about the healthy changes to come.

Learn more about the keto diet to feel more confident. Just like this book has covered so many aspects of keto, educate yourself about your diet so you can feel confident when making the decisions you need to. You'll know exactly what you can and cannot eat, which exercises you should and should not perform, and investing in some cookbooks will teach you some delicious new recipes!

Maintaining a Keto Diet

One of the hardest parts of being on the keto diet is being able to maintain and incorporate it into your lifestyle. The diet may require some tweaking if you're not losing weight as you anticipated or if you're still suffering from the flu-like "keto flu" symptoms. That is why it's very essential to have a breakdown of your macro counts to ensure you're not going over the recommended daily limit. There are many free apps you can download that will keep track of your dietary data as you input it throughout the day.

Here are some tips to help you manage a keto diet successfully in your own individual lifestyle.:

Stay hydrated! This is repeated over and over, but you'd be surprised how many people find it hard to follow. We are often so focused on eating in our diet that we forget about how important hydration is. Drinking at least 8 glasses of water is recommended for every person, but for someone on keto, your intake should be almost double that! Drinking at least half your body weight in ounces every day is a great rule of thumb to follow. For example, if you weigh 120 pounds, that's 120 / 2 = 60 ounces of water or 7.5 cups of water daily. This number should be increased depending on if you take medication, live in a humid environment, and your physical activity level. Always carry a reusable water bottle with you that you can fill easily, and set a reminder on your phone or notepad to ensure you're meeting your target.

Make sure you're getting enough salt in your diet.
Usually, with most diets, we're often urging people to reduce their salt intake to improve their health. That's because, with a normal "high" carbohydrate intake diet, the body has higher insulin levels which cause our kidneys to retain sodium. That means a higher ratio of sodium to potassium in our body. With a low-carb keto diet, the body has limited blood sugar spikes which means there's a low level of insulin in the body. The kidneys will then excrete more sodium through urination, which is one of the side effects of ketosis. That means the body's electrolyte levels are low and could result in an imbalance which can lead to symptoms like dizziness, fatigue, or muscle cramps. To counteract this, it's important that people on the keto diet include an additional 3 to 5 grams of sodium in their diet. That can be through regular iodized table salt or Himalayan pink salt which is a great alternative high in minerals. In fact, it's also high in magnesium and contains 84 essential minerals required by the human body!

Here are some other ways to add sodium to your keto diet to prevent any electrolyte imbalance:

- Be sure you're not using low-sodium broth in your cooking.
- Sprinkle Himalayan pink salt in your food throughout the day.

- Consume vegetables that are low in carbohydrates and contain sodium naturally, such as celery, cucumber, and artichokes.
- If you're having raw nuts as a snack, have a handful of the salted version to increase your sodium intake.

Try intermittent fasting. Intermittent fasting involves breaking your day into "eating" and "not eating" portions. It basically means increasing the window of time when you don't need anything, not even snacks, though you can have water, tea, and coffee to stay hydrated. It's an extra step that people can go through to see the weight loss results they want. It's especially great for people who have a habit of filling their day with unhealthy snacking! This restricts their eating window so they aren't reaching for snacks and waiting until their mealtime begins. If you wanted to do this while being on keto, it would be advisable to first have a few strong days of keto where you fill up on fat content to give you energy for your first fasting episodes.

Intermittent fasting can sound tough, but it's actually easier than you might think. You might even be participating in a 12-hour fast without knowing it! For example, if you have dinner at 8 PM and have breakfast around 8 AM the next morning, that's a 12-hour fast you've completed! All intermittent fasting does is push that window a little bit longer—to 16 hours or to 18 hours—and being cognizant of just how long your body can go without food. Most people take the added healthy eating of the keto diet and add intermittent fasting to increase their weight loss goals. For example, you may have a healthy keto-friendly dinner at night but then wait until 9 AM or 10 AM before having a keto breakfast so that you've completed a 14 to 15-hour fast.

Incorporate exercise into your routine. Exercise isn't required on the keto diet, but research shows that it's a method that can help you lose significantly more weight and lose it faster. Exercise, in general, is great for your health. It keeps your heart healthy, releases endorphins to improve your mood, keeps your limbs and muscles agile, and can help you get a good night's sleep. Sports researchers have found that high-intensity exercise can be difficult on the keto diet. That's because it activates a glucose transport chain embedded in the muscle and liver tissues called GLUT 4. This chain has receptors to seek out sugar from the circulation of bloood and store it as energy for the muscle and liver. This can be hard on a low-carbohydrate diet because you have significantly decreased your intake of carbohydrate and are no longer having such frequent blood sugar spikes due to snacking. This may impact your performance when it comes to high-intensity training like long distance running, swimming, heavy weightlifting, and sports that require a lot of energy expenditure. Some people may last in these activities for 20 or 30 seconds without a break, but the research shows your muscles will crave glucose that your body does not have and this could result in muscle cramps and injury. Research on athletes on the keto diet has shown that the keto followers tended to have slower times when it came to performing aerobic activity compared to participants not on keto.

This isn't to say you can't exercise or still have a fulfilling workout routine. It's simply about being aware of what activities you should not do in case you injure yourself. If you feel up to it, you may be able to short reps of weight lifting or high-intensity exercise, but if you overstrain your body, you will end up secreting high amounts of stress hormones which will increase your blood sugar and drive your body out of ketosis. Here are some exercises you can perform:

- Weight Training: You may still feel up to light to moderate weightlifting. As long as you are doing repetitive exercise with slight increases in weight, you will still see muscle growth on keto. Try to find a keto-friendly workout that incorporates lighter weights with higher rep counts.
- Cardio: The keto diet will give you a burst of energy to perform moderate cardio exercises. When you first start on keto and are struggling with symptoms of the keto flu, it's important you start slowly with activities

like walking and jogging. Then, you can work yourself up to moderate exercise levels depending on how energetic you feel. Some examples of cardio exercises you can perform include:

- aerobic training classes
- walking
- cycling
- short distance swimming
- jogging
- biking
- interval training classes
- recreational sports that allow for breaks

Improve your quality of sleep. If you're not sleeping well due to the changes in the keto diet, your stress hormones will be elevated, which means your blood sugar levels will increase as well. We recommend at least 7-9 hours of sleep per night, but that can depend based on your stress levels. More stress requires more sleep! dThe amount of sleep you need to feel physically and mentally alert the next day depends on your individual needs, but it's important to practice good sleeping habits and have a nighttime routine to allow your body to wind down. Here are some tips on getting a better night's sleep:

- Keep your bedroom cool, anywhere from 62-68 degrees is ideal. The colder it is, the more sleepy your body will feel to conserve energy.
- Power down screens an hour before bed. That includes TV! Instead, use the time to relax and read a book.
- Make sure your bedroom is a dark place without any distractions. Use blackout curtains if your regular curtains don't block out all the light from outside.
- Know when to stop having caffeine in the evening time so it won't interrupt your sleep cycle.
- Calm your mind through breathing exercises, meditation, or prayer. Whatever it is that helps you feel calm and able to sleep!

- Have a cup of chamomile tea or try taking over the counter melatonin, a natural supplement the body produces to help itself fall asleep.

Decrease the stress in your life. As we mentioned above when it comes to quality sleep, chronic stress can affect your body's ability to stay in ketosis and successfully burn fat. If you're going through a stressful time in your life, this might not be the best time to start the keto diet. That doesn't mean you have to eat unhealthy; it just means a more regimented diet that drastically changes what you are eating may not be healthy for you right now. When you're feeling pressured from stress factors in your life, the body secretes cortisol, the stress hormone. This can drive up your blood sugar levels, cause irritability and false hunger pangs, and weight gain. This will lower the count of ketones being produced and halt your body's ketosis process. Of course, it's easier said than done to say cure your life of all stress factors, but you can try and change how you react to these factors and give yourself some rest and relaxation. Whether it's through yoga, meditation, or breathing exercises, try and find what best helps you cope with stress.

Know how to calculate your net carbohydrates. As we've been saying over and over, restricting your carbohydrates intake is what will make all the difference about being in ketosis or not. The first step of being successful on the keto diet is knowing how to calculate your net carbs yourself. This will ensure you're not going over your daily limit and that you feel confident knowing what you can and cannot eat. The two values you need when looking at any nutrition label are: "Total Carbohydrates" and "Dietary Fiber". You simply subtract the grams of "Dietary Fiber" from grams of "Total Carbohydrates".

Total Carbs - Fiber = Net Carbs

This is the amount of net carbohydrates per serving, so you want to be aware of how many servings you have consumed. There are many calorie and carb counting apps you can download such as Cronometer or My Fitness Pal that will keep track of these values for you.

Be sure you're not eating too much protein. One of the beginner's mistake with the keto diet is making up for having no carb intake by having too much protein. But as we know, the keto diet breakdown requires only 20% protein. The majority of your caloric breakdown should be 75% fat. If you're having too much protein, then a biochemical process called gluconeogenesis occurs which turns those amino acid proteins into glucose. That's the opposite of what we want on the keto diet! It's ideal that you spread out your daily protein intake over 2 to 3 different servings throughout the day. Be sure you're not exceeding a maximum of 50 grams of protein a meal. On the other hand, you want to be sure you're not skimping on your protein intake because that can affect your muscle mass. If you're an athlete, it's a great idea to have that protein before or after a workout, either in a smoothie or a meat-rich meal. If you feel you're not losing weight as fast as you thought, you want to review your protein intake to ensure you're not going over that daily 20%.

Use MCT oil or other supplements to help your body reach ketosis. MCTs, or high-quality medium chain triglycerides, are an important addition you can make to your diet to increase your fat intake and guide your body to ketosis. These MCTs go straight to the liver and are metabolized to ketones which gives the body an instant boost of energy. You can cook with MCT oil or add it to your smoothies, coffee, and tea throughout the day. You only need a tablespoon or two and you will notice the difference! It's also important to note that recent sports research shows that muscle growth can occur 4 to 8 hours after eating protein, not right after a workout as people previously thought. That's why sports trainers have started recommending you keep having protein even after a workout instead of just before. Other substances you can incorporate into your pre or post-workout shakes include:

- Protein Powder: This is a well-known supplement that you can find in your grocery store. It's a way to increase your protein and giving you a boost of energy before your workout. It's important that you use complete protein powders such as whey or collagen.
- Exogenous Ketones: These ketones should always be paired with MCTs so they do not impair the body's ketone production. These ketones are composed of salt molecules that can provide the body with energy. In order to prevent disruption to your ketosis process, make sure you've read the instruction label and have MCTs at hand.
- Fish Oil: These supplements have become common due to recent research about how important omega-3 fatty acids. They increase brain function and protect nerve cells from damage, and also increase muscle growth. You should be having at least 1 gram of DHA and EPA fatty acids a day. That means some sort of daily fish intake. Since that can be hard to manage every day, a fish oil supplement can give you those omega-3 fatty acids.

Ensure you're not eating too many calories of fat. If you're consuming too many calories coming from fat sources, you may find yourself gaining weight instead! When you monitor your daily macro count, you should be sure your fat count is staying at 70-75%. You want to be sure you aren't ingesting too many calories as well. The number of daily calories every individual needs depends on things like age, height, size, and activity level. If you want to see a loss in weight, it's important you try to stay calorie deficit, which means you expend more calories than you intake. This can be done through exercise and an active lifestyle. If you are overweight or obese, it's even more important you maintain a lower caloric intake so you can see weight loss results. There are many free websites you can input your personal data to determine how many daily calories may be enough for you.

Common Keto Mistakes to Avoid

When talking about success on the keto diet, it's important to talk about possible pitfalls that people often land themselves. The keto diet can be a struggle for beginners so it's important you are aware of possible mistakes to avoid them. This will ensure you are eating the right macronutrient breakdown and having your body in the state of ketosis where it will readily burn fat.

Not drinking enough water. It's common knowledge that most people don't drink enough water even if they're not dieting, but water intake is very important on the keto diet. The diet naturally has diuretic effects which means you tend to urinate more to get rid of excess water weight and minerals in the body. Most experts recommend at least 1 gallon of water daily when following the keto diet. This replenishes your water intake and prevents dehydration. If you are an athlete or if you live in a humid or warm climate, you should try and drink even more water.

Being afraid of fat. We've been told all our lives that to lose weight, you want to avoid any fat in your diet. We're so used to picking the low-fat options and being wary of additional fat intake. With the keto diet, it's the complete opposite! You want to be sure your caloric fat intake is around 70-75% to ensure your body uses that fat to push itself into ketosis. These healthy fats you include in your diet are actually what keep you full and energized for longer than if you were to be getting your energy from carbohydrates. Try and buy organic or grass-fed fat items if you can budget for it so you avoid the risk of ingesting hormones.

Not enough salt intake. This is another thing we've been told to care for our health—watch your salt intake. With the keto diet, you want to carefully monitor your intake to ensure you don't feel symptoms like headaches or fatigue. As we mentioned the diuretic effects of the keto diet above, that also means the body is expelling waste in terms of minerals and sodium. That can cause a loss of electrolytes which means that you need to eat foods with sodium. Seasoning your food with a little extra salt or Himalayan salt is a great way to begin and by adding electrolytes to your water.

Eating too much dairy. Dairy can be a great complement to the keto lifestyle, but keep in mind that dairy comes with its own high caloric intake. When you pair that with protein or high fats, you may be pushing the intake of daily calories and not meeting your keto requirements. Be aware of your intake of dairy, whether that's grated cheese or full-fat Greek yogurt, to ensure it's not eating away most of your daily calories.

Not being active. The keto diet does not require exercise to lose
weight, but you can lose more weight and lose it faster when you attempt to follow an active lifestyle. If you're not incorporating some sort of physical activity in your week, be that walking, jogging, or running, then you will not see the full beneficial effects keto can have on your body. It doesn't have to be a full gym routine—even just 20 minutes of exercise two or three times a week is good!

Frequent snacking. Even though there are some keto-friendly snacks you can incorporate into your day, like Greek yogurt or low-carb fruit, frequent snacking will actually raise your blood sugar. This confuses the body regarding the old glycolysis route and knocks it out of ketosis. Try and plan your day so you eat when you are hungry and have a filling and satisfying meal that will last you until your next meal time. The more successful you are about preparing your food and menu beforehand, the less tempted you may be to reach for a snack.

Becoming stressed. Cortisol is the stress hormone the body releases when it feels you are in a stressful situation. The presence of this hormone raises your blood sugar level and knocks your body out of ketosis. You end up craving sugar and having hunger pangs, even if you aren't really hungry! If you want to have a successful keto journey, it's important you start at a time when you aren't plagued by stress. Have an outlet that helps you feel relaxed, whether that's exercise, deep breathing exercises, or meditation.

Taking cheat days. With other diets, there's often a "cheat" day involved where if you're "good" and structured about following the diet for a week, you can have a day off. But with keto, it doesn't work that way. This is a diet meant to incorporate your entire day and all your meals into a healthy lifestyle. If you feel fatigued by the diet and end up taking a cheat day, you could ruin all your hard work as your body adjusted to the low-carb intake. It's important to realize that keto is a highly involved lifestyle diet where structure and routine is important. If you want a cheat meal, you can always make yourself some delicious cheesecake or chocolate fudge fat bombs to treat yourself!

You're missing hidden carbs. Maybe you've been following keto for a few months and have become a little lax about counting carbs. This can be dangerous because sometimes, those "hidden" carbs can put you over your daily limit. And if your limit is too high, that could kick you out of ketosis and back to your body using glucose for energy. Condiments, fruit, and dairy all contain carbohydrates which you should still account for. Be sure to read the nutrition labels and account for how many servings you are consuming. Try to use healthy fats whenever you can such as olive oil instead of salad dressing or butter instead of condiments on your meat.

You're eating too much protein. Protein makes up 20% of your daily macro counts, but remember, too much protein is dangerous! The body will then store it as fat! This is exactly what you don't want on keto. Be sure you are watching your protein intake and not going over your daily 20%. Use an app to track your calories and input calories from meat and dairy. If you feel a decline in weight loss or feel keto flu symptoms return, it could be because the high protein intake has knocked your body out of ketosis.

You're not trying new foods. If you feel you're tired of the keto diet and the meals you're eating, it could be because you haven't taken the time to try new meals and types of food. Sure, there are many things you cannot eat on the keto diet, but there are many items that you can! That includes all sources of protein, many vegetables, and dairy. If you're sticking with your old meals and aren't changing it up, then you could become tired of the keto plan fast. Instead, try new recipes and ingredients and see how you like them and don't be afraid to make keto-friendly versions of ethnic cuisines. Each new ingredient has unique vitamins and minerals, and you could find a new combination you love! Don't forget that you can also make sweet, savory, or meat-loaded fat bombs which increase your fat intake and satisfy any cravings for sugar!

Stressing over your weight. As we mentioned above, stressful situations only elevate the hormones in your body which raise your blood sugar. It can be easy to feel anxious if you're not losing weight fast enough or seeing the results you want from keto quick enough. But be patient with yourself and remind yourself that your body has to adjust. It's followed the route of harnessing energy from glucose, and now it has to completely switch to ketosis! Ensure you are doing the best you can to follow your keto macro counts and eat healthy, as well as incorporating exercise into your routine and getting enough rest. Try and be patient and remember that you will gain more benefits overall the longer you last on keto.

Chapter 7: Keto Meal Prep

Meal prepping is the best way to ensure your success on the keto diet because it allows you to plan your meals (and snacks!) in advance so you aren't tempted to reach for a carb-loaded, sugary snack in a bind. Instead, you will feel secure you have keto-friendly options available for you to satisfy your hunger.

Meal prepping is successful for many reasons:

- Conquers decision fatigue: After a long and tiring day full of making decisions, the last thing you want to do is make another one about what you should eat for dinner. When you take the time to meal plan, you're reducing the amount of choices you have to make because you have a prepared meal to eat the end of the day. This ensures you don't feel frustrated and reach for something else.
- Saves time and money: At first, it seems like you're devoting a few hours to meal prepping one day of the week, but think of how much time you are saving every day when it comes to shopping, planning meals, prepping, and physically cooking. Not to mention that meal planning actually saves you money by preventing waste. You have a set portion set aside to eat, and you haven't made extras that you have to store and may eventually end up tossing out.
- Controls portions: This is always a problem if you end up making too much food and then feel like you have to eat it all or toss it out. Instead, this allows you to divide your food into portions for set days. If you're hungry after the meal, you can always have a keto-friendly snack, but you won't be overeating which results in too many calories.
- Keeps you in ketosis: The more healthy and keto-friendly meals you are planning with attention to detail like use of fat, oils, and protein, the more you are sure to stick to your keto goals. That means your

body will stay in ketosis and continue burning excess fat.

What are some simple steps to get started on your meal planning for the week? Some people may have a slightly different plan that works for them, but you want to:

First, decide what to eat. Choose a time of the week to outline your meal plan for the next seven days, including breakfast, lunch, and dinner, and any snacks or desserts if you feel you may need them. You don't have to include those for every day, but as you see they may be necessary. Have a calendar or magnetic chart that allows you to break down the recipes. Be sure that you are aware of the calorie count and how many macros are involved as well! This ensures you aren't going over your daily limit and that you are still following the rules of keto.

Know how many servings each meal will make. This way you can have a serving fresh and then store the others away for leftovers later in the week.

Make a grocery list of the ingredients you will need and be sure you have enough. Pick a day that is most convenient for you to shop for the ingredients. Remember to shop for a variety of foods that you will need but stick to your shopping list. You don't want to be tempted by low-carb or sugar-free snacks!

Cook the meals. You might prefer to do it one day or you may decide to break up the work over a few nights. Read the entire recipe before you begin and see what step will take the longest. If you need to chop your vegetables first or marinate a chicken, be sure you start with those steps so you get them out of the way. Then, you can be productive doing something else.

Once the meals are prepared, **be sure to separate them into separate containers for the week.** You don't want to mix up your portion sizes or overeat by having them all in an individual container. You can find some affordable dishwasher and microwave-safe containers online or at your local grocery store.

Items to Include In Your Meal Prep

Hard-Boiled Eggs: These are a quick and easy addition you can have to any meal. Whether it's a snack or adding on top of a salad or with a side of meat, having hard-boiled eggs ready for the week is a great way to save time. If you keep the eggs in their shells, they can stay refrigerated for up to a week.

Ground Meat: Whether it's beef, turkey, or chicken, ground meat cooks easily and can last up to 4 to 5 days in the refrigerator. You can cook it easily in a skillet with just a little bit of oil and seasoning. Be sure it's browned completely before removing from heat. This is great to add on top of tacos, salads, or as a side with hard-boiled eggs.

Cold Cut Deli Meat: Grabbing cold cuts is a great way to include in a small amount of extra flavor and protein to your lunch or breakfast. Whether it's sprinkling them in an egg omelet or adding on top of a salad, cold cuts are great with a cheese platter and olives.

Chicken: Chicken is easily prepped for meals with a quick marinade and baking it on a baking sheet until cooked through. A great way to add a little variety is to separate your chicken and use two different rubs and then bake on different sides of the same baking sheet. This gives you two flavors in the same amount of cooking time! You can pair chicken easily with vegetables or cut it up into pieces and add on top of a salad for protein. Chicken can last easily for 4 to 5 days in the fridge so you can re-heat it when you want to eat it.

Canned Tuna: This is an easy source of protein you can have on hand in your pantry. Whether you mix it with mayonnaise or mustard or add on top of a salad or pair with boiled eggs, it is a great protein and omega-3 fatty acids source. And all you need is a can opener! Once it is out of the can, you should use it within 3 to 4 days so be sure you're buying small tins that have just enough serving sizes for you.

Vegetables, Vegetables, Vegetables: Whether it's kale, cabbage, zucchini, or asparagus, there are so many vegetables you can grill or roast and have in the oven for a salad or side with your protein source. All you need is to prep these veggies, season with oil and your favorite spices, and roast in the oven as you prepare your other meal items.

4-Week Meal Prep Plan

W1 Shopping List

- Protein: 2 pounds chicken thighs, 2 cans tuna, 2 pounds salmon fillets, ground beef, salami, 1 pound shrimp
- Produce: 1 bell pepper, 3 lemons, 1 bunch of parsley, 2 cucumbers, 1 bag fresh baby spinach, 4 zucchinis, 1 head of broccoli, small package of mushrooms, avocado, blueberries
- Dairy: grated Parmesan cheese, grated cheddar cheese, 2 dozen eggs, sour cream, string cheese, unsweetened almond milk
- Dry goods: oil, raw nuts, olives

Prep:

- Chop your veggies and store in separate Ziploc bags or containers. This will make it easy for sautéing or grilling as a side or putting together a quick salad.
- Cook your ground beef.
- Chop and marinate your chicken thighs.
- Marinate your fish.
- Hard-boil a dozen eggs.

Meals:

- Monday

- Breakfast: keto-friendly coffee, mushrooms and egg omelet
- Lunch: tuna salad
- Snack: a handful of raw nuts
- Dinner: stir fry cashew chicken with sautéed broccoli

- Tuesday
  - Breakfast: spinach omelet
  - Lunch: ground beef taco salad with vegetables
  - Dinner: bake one of the marinated salmon fillets, sautéed spinach as a side

- Wednesday
  - Breakfast: avocado green smoothie with almond milk
  - Lunch: tuna salad with hard-boiled egg
  - Snack: string cheese
  - Dinner: baked chicken thighs

- Thursday
  - Breakfast: ground beef omelet
  - Lunch: keto pizza topped with spinach and cheese
  - Dinner: shrimp with zucchini noodles

- Friday
  - Breakfast: blueberry flourless pancakes
  - Lunch: hard-boiled egg salad
  - Dinner: tuna patties with vegetable stir fry

- Saturday
  - Breakfast: peanut butter almond milk smoothie
  - Lunch: shrimp salad
  - Snack: salami, cheese, and olive platter
  - Dinner: grilled salmon

- Sunday
  - Breakfast: blueberry smoothie

- Lunch: leftover grilled salmon from Saturday with vegetables
- Dinner: salmon and vegetable salad

W2 Shopping List

- Protein: 2 steaks, 1 bag shrimp, a package of bacon, 2 chicken breasts, 2 salmon fillets, scallops
- Produce: 1 bunch of parsley, 2 cucumbers, 1 bag fresh baby spinach, 1 head of broccoli, small package of mushrooms, avocado, blueberries, asparagus
- Dairy: grated Parmesan cheese, grated cheddar cheese, 2 dozen eggs, string cheese, unsweetened almond milk, sour cream

Prep:

- Chop and store your veggies.
- Marinate your steaks.
- Marinate your chicken breasts.
- Hard-boil at least a dozen eggs.
- Marinate salmon fillets.

Meals:

- Monday
  - Breakfast: classic bacon and eggs
  - Lunch: salad with fried salmon
  - Dinner: steak with side of sautéed veggies

- Tuesday
  - Breakfast: avocado smoothie
  - Lunch: salad with grated cheese and hard-boiled egg
  - Snack: a handful of blueberries
  - Dinner: scallions with asparagus

- Wednesday
  - Breakfast: healthy green smoothie

- o Lunch: cucumber and egg salad
- o Dinner: grilled salmon dinner

- Thursday
  - o Breakfast: blueberry smoothie
  - o Lunch: shrimp vegetable salad
  - o Snack: hard-boiled egg
  - o Dinner: other steak from Monday night dinner

- Friday
  - o Breakfast: omelet
  - o Lunch: veggie salad with grated cheese and any leftover shrimp from yesterday
  - o Dinner: fried salmon dinner from Wednesday night with side of veggies

- Saturday
  - o Breakfast: hard-boiled eggs and side of bacon
  - o Lunch: chicken stir fry with bell pepper and veggies
  - o Dinner: veggie salad with sour cream

- Sunday
  - o Breakfast: keto-friendly pancakes
  - o Snack: string cheese
  - o Lunch: chicken stir fry from Saturday
  - o Dinner: BLT lettuce wrap burger

W3 Shopping List

- Protein: ground beef, turkey and deli slices of meat, 2 steaks, beef, 1 pound shrimp, bacon, 2 packages of tuna
- Produce: 1 bunch of parsley, 2 cucumbers, 1 head of lettuce, 1 bag fresh baby spinach, 1 head of broccoli, raspberries, 1 head of cauliflower, avocado, blueberries, olives
- Dairy: grated Parmesan cheese, grated cheddar cheese, 2 dozen eggs, brie cheese, unsweetened almond milk

Prep:

- Hard-boil at least 10 eggs.
- Chop and store veggies.
- Cook your ground beef.
- Marinate your steaks.
- Make your cauliflower rice (or buy pre-packaged).
- Prepare half a dozen bacon, egg, and cheese muffins for breakfast.

Meals:

- Monday
  - Breakfast: omelet with veggies
  - Lunch: salad with grated cheese
  - Dinner: shrimp stir fry with cauliflower rice

- Tuesday
  - Breakfast: hard-boiled eggs and bacon
  - Lunch: brie cheese and deli meat platter with olives
  - Dinner: ground beef chili

- Wednesday
  - Breakfast: blueberry flourless pancakes
  - Lunch: tuna salad with hard-boiled egg
  - Dinner: steak with side of grilled veggies

- Thursday
  - Breakfast: bacon, cheese and egg muffins
  - Lunch: shrimp lettuce burgers
  - Dinner: keto pizza

- Friday
  - Breakfast: peanut butter smoothie
  - Lunch: leftover chili from Tuesday
  - Dinner: steak from Wed night with fresh veggies

- Saturday
    - Breakfast: bacon, cheese and egg muffins with fresh fruit
    - Lunch: bacon with side of vegetables
    - Dinner: cheese platter with olives

- Sunday
    - Breakfast: omelet with avocado smoothie
    - Lunch: tuna salad with hard-boiled egg
    - Snack: bacon, cheese and egg muffin
    - Dinner: beef stew

W4 Shopping List

- Protein: beef, chicken breasts, bacon, 1 pound salmon, salami, pork chops
- Produce: 1 head of lettuce, 4 cucumbers, 1 package of cherry tomatoes, 2 avocadoes, mushrooms, blueberries, 1 bag baby spinach, green beans
- Dairy: grated Parmesan cheese, grated cheddar cheese, cheese slices, 1 dozen eggs, unsweetened almond milk, Greek yogurt

Prep:

- Chop and store your veggies.
- Prepare egg, bacon, and cheese muffins.
- Marinate chicken breasts.
- Hard-boil eggs.
- Marinate salmon.

Meals:

- Monday
    - Breakfast: scrambled eggs
    - Lunch: beef salad
    - Dinner: grilled salmon and sautéed spinach

- Tuesday

- o Breakfast: avocado smoothie with hard-boiled egg
  - o Lunch: cheese and salami plate
  - o Dinner: cashew chicken

- Wednesday
  - o Breakfast: keto cheese rolls
  - o Lunch: salad with hard-boiled eggs
  - o Dinner: beef stew

- Thursday
  - o Breakfast: eggs with bacon
  - o Lunch: keto pizza
  - o Snack: Greek yogurt with blueberries
  - o Dinner: bacon lettuce burgers

- Friday
  - o Breakfast: flourless blueberry pancakes
  - o Lunch: mushroom and veggie omelet
  - o Dinner: pork chops with green beans

- Saturday
  - o Breakfast: egg, bacon, cheese muffin
  - o Lunch: salad with hard-boiled eggs
  - o Dinner: baked salmon with side of veggies

- Sunday
  - o Breakfast: peanut butter smoothie
  - o Lunch: salad with grated Parmesan cheese
  - o Dinner: veggie chicken soup

Chapter 8: Easy to Make Keto Recipes

Breakfast

Bacon and Eggs

Servings: 2

Nutritional Facts:
272 calories per serving
1 gram net carbs
22 grams fat
0 grams fiber
15 grams protein

Ingredients:
6-8 cherry tomatoes, halved
2-3 ounces bacon in slices
4 eggs

Directions:
1. In a small pan, fry the bacon slices until they are crispy. Set them aside on a plate.
2. In the same pan with the leftover bacon fat, fry the eggs on medium heat. Cook the eggs however you like them and add the cherry tomatoes and cook until soft.
3. Remove from heat, and then serve.

Spinach and Feta Scramble

Servings: 2

Nutritional Facts:
347 calories per serving
3 grams net carbs
16 grams protein
29 grams fat
1 gram fiber

Ingredients:
1 tablespoon heavy whipping cream
.25 cup feta cheese, crumbled
4 eggs
4 ounces fresh spinach, chopped
salt and black pepper
2 tablespoons butter
1 clove garlic, minced

Directions:
1. Mix together the eggs and heavy cream in a bowl.
2. Over medium heat, melt the butter in a skillet.
3. Then, sauté the garlic until fragrant.
4. Put the spinach in and cook until limped, then sprinkle with salt and pepper to your liking.
5. Pour the whisked eggs into the skillet and cook until set around the edges. Continue to stir until the eggs are done to your liking.
6. Remove from heat and sprinkle with the feta cheese.

Low-Carb Blueberry Pancakes

Servings: 4 (2 pancakes per serving)

Nutritional Facts:
462 calories per serving
44 grams fat
16 grams fat
7 grams net carbs
14 grams fiber

Ingredients:
3 eggs
1 teaspoon baking powder
.25 cup almond flour
.5 cup oat fiber
2 tablespoons melted butter
.25 teaspoon salt
.25 cup fresh blueberries
3 tablespoons cream cheese

Directions:
1. Mix together the cream cheese, melted butter, and the eggs in a small bowl.
2. In another bowl, combine the rest of the ingredients except for the blueberries and add that to the egg mixture. Combine until you get a smooth batter. Let it rest for 10 to 15 minutes.
3. You want to use about one third of a cup of pancake butter.
4. Fry the pancakes on medium heat in a non-stick pan.
5. Add some blueberries on top, and then flip and cook the other side. You should be able to make 8 pancakes.

Green Smoothie with Avocado and Mint

Servings: 1

Nutritional Facts:
228 calories per serving
23 grams fat
1 gram protein
1 gram fiber
5 grams carbs

Ingredients:
.5 cup almond milk
.75 cup full fat coconut milk
6-8 fresh mint leaves
a handful of ice
.5 avocado, pitted and peeled
1 tablespoon cilantro
1 teaspoon juice of lime or lemon

Directions:
1. Blend all the ingredients except the ice.
2. Once blended, add the ice and blend again.
3. Stir until you get a smooth texture.

Coconut Pancakes

Servings: 2

Nutritional Facts:
534 calories per serving
45 grams fat
18 grams protein
4 grams net carbs

Ingredients:
2 eggs
.25 teaspoon salt
.25 teaspoon ground cinnamon
3 tablespoons cream cheese
.5 tablespoon sweetener substitute, or can leave out
2 tablespoons almond flour

Directions:
1. In a bowl, mix the eggs and cream cheese.
2. Add in the sugar substitute, almond flour, salt and cinnamon powder.
3. In a pan on medium heat, add about one-third of the pancake batter and allow the pancake to brown slightly. Watch carefully to avoid any burning.
4. Flip and brown the other side and remove from heat. Do this with the rest of the batter.

Keto Cinnamon Almond Butter Smoothie

Servings: 1

Nutritional Facts:
321 calories per serving
28 grams fat
19 grams protein
10 grams carbs
5 grams fiber

Ingredients:
a handful of ice
.25 teaspoon salt
.25 teaspoon almond extract
10-12 drops Stevia sugar sweetener
.5 teaspoon ground cinnamon
1.5 unsweetened almond milk
2 tablespoons almond butter
2 tablespoons golden flax meal

Directions:
1. Add all the ingredients to the blender.
2. Stir until you get a smooth texture.

Keto Egg Muffins

Servings: 3 (2 muffins per serving)

Nutritional Facts:
332 calories per serving
27 grams fat
23 grams protein
0 grams fiber
2 grams net carbs

Ingredients:
.25 cup shredded cheese, cheddar or Parmesan
8-10 slices bacon
2 tablespoons low-carb pesto
12 eggs
2 tablespoons onion, chopped
8-10 slices salami or chorizo
salt and pepper to taste

Directions:
1. Turn on your oven and let it heat up to 350° F.
2. Then, place paper liners on your muffin tin.
3. Have your onions and salami or chorizo chopped and line it to the bottom 6 muffins.
4. In another bowl, mix the eggs, pesto, salt, pepper, and cheese until well-combined.
5. Add the egg batter to each muffin. Bake for 16-20 minutes.

Western Ham Omelet

Servings: 2

Nutritional Facts:
672 calories per serving
57 grams fat
38 grams protein
6 grams net carbs
1 gram fiber

Ingredients:
3 eggs
salt and pepper to taste
.25 onion, finely chopped
4-6 pieces deli ham, sliced
2 tablespoons butter
.25 cup shredded cheese
.25 bell pepper, finely chopped
1 tablespoon heavy whipping cream

Directions:
1. In a bowl, mix the eggs and cream then sprinkle with salt and pepper as to your liking.
2. Add in half the cheese and mix until well-combined.
3. In a frying pan on medium heat, melt your butter.
4. Sauté your chopped onions, ham, and peppers until tender.
5. Add in the egg mixture and cook until the omelet is firm.
6. Reduce the heat and add the remaining cheese and gently fold the omelet to melt the cheese. Remove from heat.

Keto Breakfast Burrito

Servings: 1

Nutritional Facts:
330 calories per serving
30 grams fat
1 grams carbs
11 grams protein

Ingredients:
2 tablespoons heavy cream
2 eggs medium
1 tablespoon butter
salt and black pepper to taste

Directions:
1. In a bowl, combine your eggs and cream and mix together.
2. In a small frying pan, add the butter and then pour in the egg mixture.
3. Place a lid over it and allow it to cook evenly.
4. Remove from heat and then add your favorite filling, any salami or vegetables.

Raspberry Avocado Smoothie

Servings: 1

Nutritional Facts:
214 calories per serving
13 grams carbs
20 grams fat
3 grams protein
8.8 grams fiber

Ingredients:
.5 avocado, peeled
.5 cup water
1 tablespoon sugar substitute
.25 cup unsweetened raspberries, fresh or frozen
2 tablespoons lemon juice
a handful of ice

Directions:
1. Add all the ingredients inside the blender.
2. Stir until smooth.

Keto Breakfast "Potatoes" Dupe

Servings: 4

Nutritional Facts:
88 calories per serving
6 grams fat
3 grams protein
4 grams net carbs

Ingredients:
3 slices bacon
1 turnip, peeled and diced
.25 onion, diced
.5 teaspoon paprika
salt and black pepper to taste
.5 garlic powder
1 green onion, sliced
1 tablespoon butter

Directions:
1. Melt the butter in a large skillet.
2. Then, sauté the turnips.
3. Sprinkle with garlic powder, salt, paprika, and black pepper.
4. In the same pan, cook the onions until tender.
5. Chop your bacon into bite-size pieces and add to the skillet and fry until golden brown.
6. Top with the green onion.

Keto No Bread Breakfast Sandwich

Servings: 2

Nutritional Facts:
345 calories per serving
20 grams protein
2 grams net carbs
0 grams fiber
30 grams fat

Ingredients:
2-3 ounces sliced cheese
salt and pepper to taste
2 ounce smoked deli ham
4 eggs
2 tablespoon butter

Directions:
1. In a small frying pan, fry the eggs to your preference using the butter, then sprinkle with salt and pepper. You want an egg to be the "base" of your sandwich.
2. Then, place the ham and cheese layers.
3. Top off the meat layers with another egg "bread" slice on top.
4. If you want the cheese to slightly melt, you can assemble this in the pan so it melts the cheese.

Keto Mushroom Omelet

Servings: 1

Nutritional Facts:
500 calories per serving
25 grams protein
41 grams fat
1 gram fiber
4 gram net carbs

Ingredients:
salt and black pepper to taste
3 mushrooms, chopped
3 tablespoons onion, minced
1 tablespoon shredded cheese
1 tablespoon butter
3 eggs

Directions:
1. In a bowl, whisk the eggs then sprinkle with salt and pepper seasoning.
2. In a small skillet, melt the butter over medium heat.
3. Pour the egg mixture into the skillet.
4. Once the eggs begin to cook and get firm, sprinkle the mushrooms, onion, and cheese on top.
5. Once edges begin to crinkle, fold it in half and let the cheese melt a little.
6. Remove from heat, then serve.

Lunch

Lamb Kebabs

Servings: 2 (2 meatballs per serving)

Nutritional Facts:
318 calories per serving
20 grams protein
0 grams carbs
26 grams fat
0 grams fiber

Ingredients:
.25 cup fresh parsley, chopped
1 teaspoon paprika
.5 teaspoon sea salt
.5 pound grass-fed ground lamb
1 teaspoon lemon juice

Directions:
1. Let your oven heat up to 300° F.
2. In a food processor, add all the ingredients and allow for them to be evenly mixed.
3. Remove the mixture and form into kebab forms on skewers or you can make into 2" round meatballs.
4. Bake 20-23 minutes until the meat is cooked through.
5. Garnish with additional parsley if you prefer.

Zucchini Noodles and Shrimp

Servings: 4

Nutritional Facts:
231 calories per serving
16 grams fat
17 grams protein
2 grams fiber
9 grams carbs

Ingredients:
1 pound medium shrimp, peeled
3-4 cloves garlic, minced
.5 teaspoon red pepper flakes
2 tablespoons lemon or lime juice
1.5 pounds zucchini noodles
3 tablespoons grated Parmesan cheese
.25 cup vegetable stock
2 tablespoons butter
salt and black pepper to taste

Directions:
1. In a large skillet over medium heat, sauté your garlic in butter
2. Then, add in the shrimp.
3. To taste, sprinkle with black pepper, red pepper flakes, and salt.
4. Stir and cook the shrimp until no longer raw.
5. Stir in the juice of lemon and the vegetable stock, then season with additional salt and pepper as to your liking.
6. In the same pane, cook the zucchini noodles until tender for about 2-3 minutes.
7. Garnish with Parmesan before serving.

Low-Carb Chili in the Crock Pot

Servings: 4

Nutritional Facts:
310 calories per serving
18 grams fat
22 grams protein
13 grams carbs
3 grams fiber

Ingredients:
.5 cup tomato sauce
1 tablespoon butter
1 pound ground beef
1 tablespoon Worcestershire sauce
1 teaspoon chili powder
1 teaspoon dried oregano
3 cloves garlic, minced
.5 onion, chopped
1 teaspoon black pepper
1 teaspoon sea salt
1 tablespoon cumin powder

Directions:
1. In a skillet over medium heat, sauté the onions in butter until golden brown.
2. Then, add in the garlic and ground beef. Cook for 10-12 minutes until the meat has browned.
3. Transfer this beef to your slow cooker.
4. Add in the pot the remaining ingredients and spices and stir until well-combined.
5. Based on how quickly you want the dish done, you can cook for 6-8 hours on low or 3-4 hours on high.

Low-Carb Taco Salad

Servings: 4

Nutritional Facts:
245 calories per serving
7 grams carbs
22 grams protein
14 grams fat
2.4 grams fiber

Ingredients:
.5 pound ground beef
8-10 cherry tomatoes, halved
.25 cup shredded cheddar cheese
.25 cup red onion, chopped
1 tablespoon cilantro
3 tablespoons sour cream
.5 peeled avocado, diced
1.5 cup lettuce, chopped
1 teaspoon red chili powder
.5 teaspoon garlic powder
.5 teaspoon sea salt
.5 teaspoon cumin powder
.5 teaspoon dried oregano

Directions:
1. Combine all your spices in a bowl and stir until well-incorporated.
2. Cook your ground beef in a skillet over medium heat until browned and cooked through.
3. Add in to your spice bowl and then add the taco seasoning you prepared.
4. Combine the rest of the vegetables, cheese, and sour cream.
5. Top with cilantro, then serve.

Low-Carb Keto Chili

Servings: 6 (1 cup per serving)

Nutritional Facts:
362 calories per serving
23 grams fat
7 grams carbs
35 grams protein

Ingredients:
2 tablespoons butter
2 stalks celery, chopped
1 15 ounce can of tomato sauce
1 16 ounce can of beef broth
1 teaspoon black pepper
1 teaspoon garlic powder
1 tablespoon cumin powder
1 teaspoon salt
1 teaspoon chili powder
2 pounds ground beef
1 teaspoon chipotle powder

Directions:
1. In a large pot, cook the celery in butter until soft.
2. Stir in the beef and the spices until well-combined.
3. Then, pour in the tomato sauce and the broth and let it simmer for 12-15 minutes. Stir until well-incorporated.
4. Let it simmer and allow the liquid to slightly reduce, then serve.

Avocado, Chicken, and Cucumber Salad

Servings: 3

Nutritional Facts:
534 calories per serving
10 grams carbs
5 grams fiber
38 grams fat
40 grams protein

Ingredients:
.25 red onion, chopped
1 tablespoon lemon or lime juice
1 peeled avocado, diced
salt and black pepper to taste
2-3 small tomatoes, chopped
1 large cucumber, chopped
2 tablespoons olive oil
.5 Rotisserie chicken, shredded

Directions:
1. In a large bowl, mix your onion, avocado, chicken, cucumber, and tomatoes.
2. Sprinkle with black pepper and salt as to your liking.
3. Pour in your lemon juice and olive oil.
4. Toss until everything is well-combined.

Avocado Egg Salad

Servings: 6

Nutritional Facts:
168 calories per serving
6 grams carbs
12 grams fat
8 grams protein
3 grams fiber

Ingredients:
2 tablespoons lemon or lime juice
.25 red onion, finely chopped
2 teaspoons parsley, chopped
.5 teaspoon salt
.5 teaspoon black pepper
2 peeled avocadoes, diced
6 hard-boiled eggs

Directions:
1. Peel then roughly chop the hard-boiled eggs.
2. Add to a mixing bowl along with the avocado and stir well. The avocado becomes creamier the more you stir.
3. Add the lemon juice and onion.
4. Add in the salt and black pepper.
5. Sprinkle with parsley, then serve immediately.

Keto Cabbage Soup

Servings: 5

Nutritional Facts:
264 calories per serving
17 grams protein
18 grams fat
2 grams fiber
6 grams carbs

Ingredients:
1 can diced tomatoes (6 oz.)
2 cups water
salt and black pepper to taste
.5 head large cabbage, chopped
1 clove garlic, minced
1 teaspoon cumin powder
1 pound ground beef
.5 onion, diced
1 tablespoon butter

Directions:
1. In a large pan on medium heat, cook the ground beef in butter. Allow it to cook through.
2. Then, add in the onion and stir to cook.
3. Then, transfer the onion and beef mixture to a large pot.
4. Pour in the water and add all the other ingredients. Sprinkle with salt and black pepper to your taste.
5. Lower the heat and simmer for 30-40 minutes until the soup has thickened.

BLT Lettuce Wraps

Servings: 2

Nutritional Facts:
168 calories per serving
8 grams carbs
11 grams protein
2 grams fiber
10 grams fat

Ingredients:
3 large iceberg lettuce leaves
1 tomato, diced
4-6 slices bacon
1 tablespoon light mayonnaise
salt and black pepper to taste
1 tablespoon butter

Directions:
1. Lay out 2 leaves of the lettuce and shred the third leaf which will be used as a topping.
2. In a pan over medium heat, fry the bacon slices in butter until golden brown.
3. Roughly chop the bacon into small pieces once cool.
4. Combine the mayonnaise, shredded lettuce, and tomato in a small bowl, seasoning with salt and pepper.
5. Divide the mixture on 2 lettuce wraps and then eat as a wrap.

Stuffed Peppers with Greek Yogurt Chicken Salad

Servings: 6

Nutritional Facts:
118 calories per serving
3 grams fat
16 grams carbs
8 grams protein

Ingredients:
.5 cucumber, diced
.5 cup cherry tomatoes, halved
2 cups chicken, cooked and shredded
1 teaspoon salt
1 tablespoon mustard
1 teaspoon black pepper
.75 cup Greek yogurt
.5 cup celery, diced
3 bell peppers, halved and de-seeded
1 tablespoon fresh parsley, chopped

Directions:
1. Mix the Greek yogurt and mustard in large salad bowl.
2. Sprinkle with salt and pepper to your liking.
3. Add celery, chicken, tomatoes, and cucumbers to the yogurt. Stir well to combine.
4. Divide the mixture into each of the bell pepper boats.
5. Garnish with fresh parsley before serving.

Keto Pizza

Servings: 2

Nutritional Facts:
1053 calories per serving
90 grams fat
44 grams protein
8 grams carbs
2 grams fiber

Ingredients:
Crust
.75 cup shredded mozzarella cheese
4 eggs
Toppings
3 tablespoons low-carb tomato sauce
.5 cup shredded mozzarella cheese
8-10 slices pepperoni
3-4 pitted olives, sliced
1 teaspoon dried oregano

Directions:
1. Let your oven heat up to 400° F.
2. To make the crust, mix the eggs and cheese. Stir until well-combined.
3. Spread out the egg and cheese batter on a baking tray. You can make 2 circular pizzas.
4. Bake for 12-14 minutes until the crust turns light brown. Remove from heat and let cool.
5. Re-set your oven temperature to 450° F.
6. Add the toppings to the pizza with the tomato paste first, then sprinkling with cheese, pepperoni, olives, and oregano.
7. Return it to the oven for another 6-10 minutes until the pizza cheese has cooked.

Keto Tuna Salad

Servings: 1

Nutritional Facts:
993 calories per serving
6 grams net carbs
92 grams fat
32 grams protein
5 grams fiber

Ingredients:
1 tablespoon olive oil
2 hard-boiled eggs
.5 teaspoon lemon juice
.5 cup lettuce, chopped
4-5 cherry tomatoes, halved
.5 teaspoon mustard
.3 cup mayonnaise
2.5 ounce tuna
1 celery stalk, chopped
salt and pepper to taste

Directions:
1. Combine your tuna, mustard, lemon juice, mayonnaise, and celery in a large bowl.
2. Sprinkle with salt and black pepper to taste.
3. Place the tuna mixture on the lettuce.
4. Slice the hard-boiled eggs and put on top of the salad.
5. Then, add in the tomatoes, and olive oil as dressing.

Keto Brie Cheese and Salami Plate

Servings: 2

Nutritional Facts:
1143 calories per serving
5 grams net carbs
102 grams fat,
38 grams protein
10 grams fiber

Ingredients:
1 avocado, peeled and sliced
.25 cup olive oil
.5 cup macadamia nuts
.5 cup salami
.25 cup lettuce, chopped
.5 ounce Brie cheese

Directions:
1. Arrange the avocado slices, nuts, lettuce, salami, and cheese on a plate.
2. Drizzle with olive oil and serve.

Dinner

Shrimp Avocado Salad with Feta Cheese

Servings: 2

Nutritional Facts:
422 calories per serving
6 grams fiber
12 grams carbs
33 grams fat

21 grams protein

Ingredients:
1 tablespoon lemon juice
2 tablespoons butter, melted
.3 cup fresh parsley, chopped
1 small tomato, diced
1 avocado, diced
1 tablespoon olive oil
.5 teaspoon black pepper
8 ounces shrimp, peeled
.3 cup feta cheese, crumbled
.5 teaspoon salt

Directions:
1. Mix together the shrimp with the melted butter in a small bowl until coated.
2. In a large pan, cook the shrimp over medium heat.
3. Once cooked, remove from heat and let cool in a place.
4. Add all the other ingredients in a large bowl except the olive oil and toss together to mix.
5. Add the shrimp and stir until everything well-combined.
6. Drizzle with the olive oil and sprinkle with some salt and pepper, then serve.

Chicken Fajita Lettuce Wraps

Servings: 2

Nutritional Facts:
483 calories per serving
35 grams fat
12 grams carbs
4 grams fiber
20 grams protein

Ingredients:
.5 teaspoon salt
1 teaspoon chili powder
.5 teaspoon cumin powder
.5 teaspoon garlic powder
.5 teaspoon black pepper
2 tablespoons butter
2 tablespoons lemon or lime juice
2 large leaves of iceberg lettuce
1 avocado, peeled and sliced
.5 red onion, sliced
.5 bell pepper, sliced
1 chicken breast, diced

Directions:
1. Combine all the spices for the fajita seasoning in a small bowl. Set aside.
2. In another bowl, add your chicken chunks and marinate it with the olive oil, lemon juice, and 3-4 tablespoons of the seasoning you just mixed together.
3. In a large pan, cook the onion and bell pepper in butter in a large pan on medium heat.
4. Season with some of the fajita seasoning and then remove from heat once hot. Set aside.
5. Add in the chicken to the pan.
6. When cooked through, add the vegetables back to the pan and combine everything. Remove from heat.
7. Assemble these on your lettuce wraps and top with avocado.

Garlic Butter Baked Salmon

Servings: 3

Nutritional Facts:
275 calories per serving
31 grams protein
2 grams carbs
14 grams fat
0.3 grams fiber

Ingredients:
2 tablespoons lemon juice
.5 teaspoon black pepper
.5 teaspoon red pepper flakes
.5 teaspoon salt
1 tablespoon parsley, chopped
2 tablespoons butter
1 pound salmon, cut into 3 portions
3 cloves garlic, minced

Directions:
1. Let your oven heat up to 375° F.
2. In a saucepan, sauté the garlic in butter on medium heat until fragrant.
3. Turn off the heat before it burns.
4. Place your salmon pieces in individual pieces of foil that you can wrap around them.
5. On one side, use a brush to spread the garlic butter sauce over each piece of salmon.
6. Then, sprinkle it with the salt, red pepper flakes, and black pepper.
7. Use the foil to cover each piece so the sauce does not leak. Bake for 12-15 minutes until firm.
8. You can place under the broiler for another few minutes to add more crisp.
9. Remove from heat, then serve.

Zucchini Pizza Slices

Servings: 2

Nutritional Facts:
382 calories per serving
27 grams fat
13 grams carbs
33 grams protein

Ingredients:
1 teaspoon fresh basil, chopped
.5 teaspoon red chili flakes
1 cup shredded mozzarella cheese
.5 onion, diced
.25 bell pepper, diced
3-4 mushrooms, sliced
.5 can of low-carb pizza sauce
2 zucchini slices, sliced lengthwise

Directions:
1. Let your oven heat up to 400° F.
2. Scoop out the flesh and seeds of the halved zucchini.
3. Spread each zucchini boat with the pizza sauce.
4. Then, top with cheese, onion, mushrooms, bell pepper, and basil.
5. Place on a baking tray and bake for 12-14 minutes or until the cheese is melted.
6. Remove from oven and top with red chili flakes.

Keto Shrimp Scampi

Servings: 2

Nutritional Facts:
362 calories per serving
7 grams carbs
48 grams protein
15 grams fat
2 grams fiber

Ingredients:
2 tablespoons lemon juice
1 pound shrimp, peeled
.5 teaspoon red pepper flakes
.75 pound squash noodles
2 tablespoons butter
.25 cup chicken broth
salt and black pepper to taste

Directions:
1. Use a spiralizer to form your squash noodles. You can also buy pre-packaged and add that nutritional data.
2. On medium heat, add in the butter in a frying pan. Allow it to melt.
3. Then, add the lemon juice, chicken broth, and allow it to boil.
4. Add the shrimp.
5. Then, season with salt, red pepper flakes, and black pepper.
6. Lower the heat and allow the shrimp to simmer until they are cooked through.
7. Add in the noodles to the pan and coat in the sauce.
8. Mix it to combined well with the shrimp.
9. Remove from heat and serve.

One Pan Pesto Chicken with Veggies

Servings: 2

Nutritional Facts:
422 calories per serving
22 grams protein
12 grams carbs
32 grams fat
4 grams fiber

Ingredients:
2 tablespoons butter
3 tablespoons pesto
.5 cup cherry tomatoes, halved
.5 pound asparagus, halved and ends trimmed
1 small tomato, diced
.5 pound chicken thighs, sliced into strips
1 teaspoon black pepper
1 teaspoon paprika
1 teaspoon salt

Directions:
1. In a large skillet, add in the butter. Allow it to melt.
2. Then, add your sliced chicken thighs and season with the spices.
3. Add the chopped tomatoes and cook until the chicken is cooked through.
4. Remove the chicken thighs from heat.
5. In the same pan, add in the asparagus and sprinkle with additional salt.
6. Over medium heat, cook for 5-10 minutes until tender.
7. Add the pesto and chicken back to the skillet and re-heat.
8. Remove from heat and serve.

Brazilian Garlic Steak

Servings: 4

Nutritional Facts:
432 calories per serving
32 grams fat
1 grams carbs
39 grams protein

Ingredients:
1 teaspoon salt
4 cloves garlic, minced
.5 teaspoon black pepper
1 teaspoon paprika
4 tablespoons butter, divided
1.5 pound skirt steak, cut into 4 pieces

Directions:
1. Pat your steak dry to avoid having any moisture.
2. Season each side with salt, paprika, and black pepper.
3. In a skillet, brown each side of the steak in melted butter for 3-5 minutes on each side. Transfer to a plate.
4. In the same skillet, add the rest of the butter and add the minced garlic. Allow it to become lightly golden brown and fragrant.
5. Sprinkle with salt for taste.
6. Pour on top of the steak pieces and garnish with parsley before serving.

Cashew Chicken

Servings: 3

Nutritional Facts:
331 calories per serving
8 grams carbs
23 grams protein
24 grams fat
1.2 grams fiber

Ingredients:
.5 bell pepper, diced
3 cloves garlic, minced
.25 onion, diced
1 tablespoon sesame seeds
1 tablespoon vinegar
1 tablespoon ginger, minced
2 tablespoons butter
.5 tablespoon chili sauce
.25 cup raw cashews
.5 teaspoon salt
3 boneless chicken thighs, cubed
.5 teaspoon paprika

Directions:
1. In a frying pan on low heat, lightly dry toast your cashews until golden brown. Set aside.
2. Increase the heat and add the butter to the pan.
3. Once melted, add the garlic and ginger.
4. Once fragrant, add in the chicken cubes until cooked through.
5. Add in the diced onion and bell pepper. Cook until tender.
6. Then, pour in vinegar and chili sauce, then season with salt and paprika.
7. Garnish with the cashews and sesame seeds.
8. Remove from heat when there is no excess liquid in the pan. Serve.

Garlic Scallops

Servings: 2

Nutritional Facts:
389 calories per serving
7 grams carbs
25 grams protein
18 grams fat
1 gram fiber

Ingredients:
.25 cup butter, melted
2 tablespoons lemon juice
.5 teaspoon salt
6 cloves garlic, minced
1 teaspoon lemon zest
.5 teaspoon red pepper flakes
.5 teaspoon black pepper
.25 cup fresh parsley, chopped
1 pound scallops

Directions:
1. Make sure your scallops are dry with no additional moisture.
2. In a large cast iron skillet, add just a drizzle of the melted butter to coat the pan.
3. Sear the scallops, seasoning with salt, red pepper flakes, and black pepper, for 5-8 minutes until cooked through.
4. Then, add the rest of the butter and add the garlic.
5. Add the lemon juice and zest.
6. Remove from heat once the moisture has been cooked away.
7. Garnish with the parsley before serving.

Parmesan Coated Boneless Pork Chops

Servings: 2

Nutritional Facts:
342 calories per serving
21 grams fat
1 gram carbs
38 grams protein

Ingredients:
4 boneless pork chops
1 teaspoon paprika
2 tablespoons butter
salt and black pepper to taste
Low-Carb Crust
1 egg, beaten
a pinch of lemon zest
1 tablespoon fresh parsley, chopped
.25 cup pork rinds, crushed
.25 cup grated Parmesan cheese
1 clove garlic, minced

Directions:
1. Make sure your pork chops are at room temperature. Using a paper towel, pat it dry.
2. Sprinkle generously with salt, paprika, black pepper.
3. To make the low-carb crust, put all the cheese, pork rinds, parsley, garlic and lemon zest in a plate. Mix well so it's well-combined.
4. Then, beat the egg in a small bowl.
5. In a large frying pan, add the butter until it is melted.
6. Then, dip each pork chop in the coating and flip it over to ensure it's well covered.
7. Then, dip it in the egg mixture and let any extra egg run off before dipping again in the cheese mixture.
8. Put the coated pork chop to the pan and let it cook for 3-4 minutes until cooked through.
9. Turn and cook the other side. Do the same for the remaining pork chops.

10. Let rest for 8-10 minutes, then serve.

Keto Ground Beef Plate

Servings: 2

Nutritional Facts:
904 calories per serving
78 grams fat
48 grams protein
1 gram fiber
5 grams net carbs

Ingredients:
.5 cucumber, diced
.5 bell pepper, diced
2 tablespoons olive oil
.25 cup shredded cheddar cheese
2 tablespoons butter
.25 cup lettuce, chopped
.75 pound ground beef
salt and black pepper to taste

Directions:
1. Cook the ground beef in butter in a frying pan over medium heat. Let it cook through.
2. Sprinkle with some salt and pepper for seasoning.
3. Once cooked, remove from the heat and combine with the raw vegetables and cheese.
4. Serve with olive oil.

Keto No Noodle Chicken Soup

Servings: 4

Nutritional Facts:
502 calories per serving
40 grams fat
32 grams protein
1 gram fiber
4 gram net carbs

Ingredients:
1 celery stalk, chopped
.5 teaspoon black pepper
4 cups chicken broth
1 clove garlic, minced
1 small onion, minced
1 tablespoon fresh parsley, chopped
.5 teaspoon salt
.5 carrot, chopped
.75 Rotisserie chicken, shredded
1 cup cabbage, sliced
3-4 mushrooms, chopped
4 tablespoons butter

Directions:
1. In a large pot, sauté in butter the celery, mushroom, onions, and garlic. Let it cook for a few minutes until the garlic is fragrant.
2. Then, add the carrot, parsley, and chicken broth.
3. Sprinkle with some salt and pepper for seasoning.
4. Simmer the broth until the vegetables become tender.
5. Now, add in the chicken and the cabbage.
6. Simmer again for 12-15 minutes until the cabbage becomes tender.

Keto Baked Salmon

Servings: 3

Nutritional Facts:
563 calories per serving
49 grams fat
31 grams protein
0 grams fiber
1 gram net carbs

Ingredients:
2 tablespoons lemon juice
.5 lemon, sliced
1 pound salmon
.5 teaspoon ground black pepper
2 tablespoons butter
.5 teaspoon salt

Directions:
1. Let your oven heat up to 400° F.
2. Sprinkle your salmon with salt and black pepper for some seasoning and place on a baking tray.
3. Slice the lemon into thin slices and place on top of the salmon. Also drizzle the fish with lemon juice.
4. Bake for about 25-35 minutes until the fish is flaky.
5. Add the tablespoons of butter on top and allow it to melt, then serve.

Dessert

Keto Flourless Cake

Servings: 12

Nutritional Facts:
293 calories per serving
16 grams protein
8 grams carbs
27 grams fat
4.5 grams fiber

Ingredients:
.6 cup butter or ghee
4 eggs
1 cup boiling water
.5 cup low-carb sweetener substitute
12 ounces unsweetened baking chocolate
.25 teaspoon salt
.3 cup water

Directions:
1. Line a 9" pan with parchment.
2. In a small pot, heat the water, salt, and the sugar sweetener until the salt and sweetener are dissolved.
3. Melt the baking chocolate in the microwave or using a double broiler method.
4. Mix the butter and chocolate in a large bowl.
5. Pour in the hot water and add in one egg at a time, while beating after each one.
6. Then, pour the mixture into the pan and wrap the outside with foil.
7. Place the pan in a larger cake pan and add the boiling water to the outside.
8. Bake for about 45 minutes at 350° F.
9. Chill the cake overnight in the fridge.

Peanut Butter Milkshake

Servings: 1

Nutritional Facts:
253 calories per serving
13 grams carb
4 grams fiber
6 grams fat
36 grams protein

Ingredients:
a handful of ice
1 teaspoon vanilla extract
2 tablespoons collagen powder
2 tablespoons substitute sweetener
3 tablespoons peanut butter
.5 cup unsweetened almond milk
.5 cup cottage cheese

Directions:
1. In a blender, put all the ingredients together.
2. Stir until the mixture is smooth.

Chocolate Peanut Butter Cups

Servings: 12

Nutritional Facts:
148 calories per serving
3.18 grams protein
8 grams carbs
3.3 grams fiber
13.4 grams fat

Ingredients:
6 ounces sugar-free dark chocolate
1 tablespoon cocoa butter
Peanut Butter filling
.5 teaspoon vanilla extract
.25 cup substitute sugar sweetener
2 tablespoons butter
.5 cup peanut butter

Directions:
1. Line a muffin tin with silicone or paper liners.
2. In a microwaveable bowl, melt the dark chocolate and mix with the cocoa butter until there are no lumps and it's smooth.
3. Add about half the chocolate into 12 of the liners.
4. Refrigerate for 10-15 minutes until hard.
5. In another microwavable bowl, melt the butter and peanut butter and mix with the sweetener and vanilla extract.
6. Divide into 12 portions add some to each paper cup liner.
7. Refrigerate for another 10 minutes until hardened.
8. Then, add the rest of the chocolate on top to form a last top layer.
9. Refrigerate again for 15-20 minutes until frozen solid.

Lemon Fat Bombs

Servings: 16

Nutritional Facts:
3 grams total carbs
12 grams fat
0.8 grams protein
2.1 grams fiber

Ingredients:
.25 cup coconut oil
1-2 tablespoons lemon zest and lemon extract
15-20 drops Stevia sugar sweetener
7 ounces coconut butter

Directions:
1. Your coconut butter oil should be softened at room temperature.
2. Zest your lemon.
3. In a bowl, mix all the ingredients together and be sure it's well-combined.
4. Line a muffin tray with liners and pour about 1 tablespoon to the coconut mixture into each liner.
5. Refrigerate for 30-60 minutes until solid.

Keto Chocolate Fudge

Servings: 10

Nutritional Facts:
152 calories per serving
12 grams fat
4 grams carbs
2 grams net carbs
2 grams fiber

Ingredients:
4 ounces dark chocolate
.75 cup coconut butter
1 teaspoon vanilla extract
4-7 drops artificial sugar sweetener

Directions:
1. In a microwave-safe bowl or using the double broiler method, melt the chocolate and coconut butter.
2. Add the vanilla and sweetener to your taste.
3. Now, pour the mixture into a baking sheet lined with parchment paper.
4. Refrigerate for 60 minutes or until the mixture has hardened.
5. Cut into 10-12 pieces.

Vanilla Cheesecake Bombs

Servings: 12

Nutritional Facts:
94 calories per serving
10 grams fat
2 grams fiber
4 grams carbs
2 grams net carbs

Ingredients:
1 package of cream cheese (8 oz.)
.75 cup heavy cream, divided into 2 portions
.5 cup substitute sugar sweetener
1.5 teaspoon vanilla extract

Directions:
1. Mix together the vanilla extract, sugar sweetener, and cream cheese together in a large bowl.
2. A hand mixture will give you an even texture and be sure to scrape the bowl so all the ingredients mix together.
3. Add half the heavy cream to the bowl.
4. Let the bowl rest for 5-10 minutes so the sugar can dissolve.
5. Then, add the second half of the heavy cream and mix until there are sharp peaks at the top.
6. Have a muffin tray ready lined with paper or silicone liners.
7. Use a tablespoon or cookie scoop to scoop evenly into each mixture.
8. Refrigerate for 60 minutes or until mixture hardens.

Raw Nuts and Raspberry Chocolate Bark

Servings: 8-10

Nutritional Facts:
84 calories per serving
1.8 grams fiber
3.2 grams carbs
8 grams fat

Ingredients:
.5 cup coconut butter
.25 cup raw walnuts, unsalted
.5 cup raspberries, fresh or frozen
.25 cup raw almonds, unsalted
1 tablespoon unsweetened cocoa powder
2 teaspoons substitute sugar sweetener
.25 cup almond butter

Directions:
1. First, roughly chop your nuts until they are in bite-size pieces.
2. Then, combine the almond and nut butter, sugar, and cocoa powder in a bowl.
3. Spread out the mixture on a parchment lined baking sheet.
4. Ensure your raspberries are soft and microwave them for 15-25 seconds until the fruit is soft and releasing juices.
5. Add the raw nuts and raspberries to the chocolate.
6. Refrigerate the tray for 60 minutes or until it hardens.
7. Cut into 8-10 pieces.

Conclusion

Thanks for making it through to the end of *Ketogenic Diet*. We hope this book was informative and able to provide you with all the answers you had regarding the ketogenic diet.

This is a diet that has gained so much popularity in recent years but it can be a bit overwhelming for beginners. That's because rather than just a simple list of what you can and cannot keto, the keto diet is more specific with its daily caloric breakdown. With 75% fat, 20% protein, and ~5% carbohydrate intake, the diet aims to train the body to adjust to the reduced carbohydrate intake and take the body on the ketosis pathway to harness energy. This produces more energy-rich ketones that people feel help their mental acuity and gives them more daily energy.

The keto diet requires some research on what you can and cannot eat and understanding how daily calories are calculated. There are many things you can eat, along with protein, vegetables, fruit, and dairy, but it's important to be aware of each item's caloric breakdown and count that towards your daily numbers. Using an app or a website that keeps track of your food intake is a great way to hold yourself accountable and begin to notice if your body has achieved ketosis. Though there may be a "slump" as your body adjusts and you feel symptoms of the "keto flu", remind yourself that it's only temporary and that your new diet has many positive health benefits.

Whether you're hoping to reduce your risk of diabetes, lower your blood pressure, gain more focus and mental acuity in your work, or simply hope to lose weight you haven't been able to get rid of, it's important you stay motivated regarding your goals to help you through the adjustment phase. The side effects are temporary, and it's important that you mold your lifestyle to adjust around them, such as incorporating exercise into your week, getting enough sleep, avoiding stress, and ensuring you're staying hydrated.

With more than 30 keto-friendly recipes in this book for breakfast, lunch, dinner, and dessert, we can help you plan your shopping list and meal prep for your week. Meal prepping can save you time, money, and energy when it comes to having a keto-friendly meal ready at the end of the day. This makes it less likely you're tempted to break your diet and ruin your day of healthy eating!

The more you've learned about keto, the more comfortable you will feel making decisions about what you can and cannot eat. We've included a detailed shopping list on each category of items you can shop for with net carbohydrate counts so you can decide which fruits and vegetables are important to you. You can even have a keto dessert as long as you're aware of the calories you're eating and how it adds to your daily count. If you're eating too much fat or too much protein, it could negatively impact your state of ketosis and result in you gaining weight instead.

Your success on the keto diet depends on a lot of factors, even simple ones such as staying hydrated and achieving a balance in electrolytes. We've included many tips on how you can make your keto diet a successful journey and gain the most benefits as long as you incorporate an active lifestyle and be aware of hidden carbs in things like fruit, alcohol, and condiments. By avoiding common pitfalls, you can feel confident that you can harness success on keto and meet your weight loss and health goals.

If you've found this book helpful toward your keto journey, we would appreciate a review!

17569967R00072

Printed in Great Britain
by Amazon